Towards Neurobioethics

Towards Neurobioethics

By

Darlei Dall'Agnol

Cambridge Scholars Publishing

Towards Neurobioethics

By Darlei Dall'Agnol

This book first published 2020

Cambridge Scholars Publishing

Lady Stephenson Library, Newcastle upon Tyne, NE6 2PA, UK

British Library Cataloguing in Publication Data
A catalogue record for this book is available from the British Library

ISBN (10): 1-5275-5801-0
ISBN (13): 978-1-5275-5801-4

To Fred, Peter and Steve

CONTENTS

ABBREVIATIONS

ADD	Attention Deficit Disorder
ADHD	Attention Deficit-HyperactivityDisorder
ANVISA	Agência Nacional de Vigilância Sanitária (BR)
APA	American Psychiatric Association
BCIs	Brain-Computer Interfaces
B.R.A.I.N. Initiative	Brain Research through Advancing Innovative Neurotechnologies
CBA	Cost-Benefits Analysis
CEA	Cost-effectiveness Analysis
CNS	Central Nervous System
DBS	Deep Brain Stimulation
DIY tDCS	(Do It Yourself) Transcranial Direct Current Stimulation
DLPFC	Dorsolateral Prefrontal Cortex
DSM-V	Diagnostic and Statistical Manual of Mental Disorders
ICD	International Classification of Diseases
IRBs	Institutional Review Boards
FDA	Food and Drug Administration
FEP	First Ethical Principle
fMRI	Functional Magnetic Resonance Imaging
MR	Magnetic Rosonance
O3	Our Brain, Our Selves, Our World: An International Research Consortium on Neuroscience, Ethics and Society
PCE	Pharmaceutical Cognitive Enhancers (PCE)
PET	Positron Emission Tomography
PFC	Prefrontal Cortex
RTW	Rational Theory of Welfare
tDCS	Transcranial Direct Current Stimulation
TMS	Transcranial Magnetic Stimulation
UDHR	Universal Declaration of Human Rights
VMPFC	Ventromedial Prefontal Cortex
WM	Working Memory

Some Philosophical Works (see references):

NE	*Nicomachean Ethics* (Aristotle)
GMM	*Groundwork of the Metaphysics of Morals* (Kant)
TLP	*Tractatus Logico-philosophicus* (Wittgenstein)
PE	*Principia Ethica* (Moore)
PI	*Philosophical Investigations* (Wittgenstein)
UTIL	*Utilitarianism* (Mill)

ACKNOWLEDGMENTS

In the first semester of the academic year 2017-8, I presented a three-part lecture series entitled "Respectful Care in Bioethics and Neuroethics," co-sponsored by the Department of Philosophy and the Center for Ethics and Humanities in the Life Sciences, at the Michigan State University in East Lansing, US. For the lectures, I used my paper "Knowing-how to care" and my book "Care and Respect in Bioethics" (see References) as the main bibliographical sources. At this time, I also did some research on the foundations of neuroethics to investigate the practical implications of the concept of *caring respect.* This book is a revised version of those lectures, which I delivered as a Visiting Scholar supported by the Fulbright Foundation. Thus, I am grateful to Fulbright for funding this challenging journey and for their work to improve the academic relationship between Brazil and the US.

I would also like to thank the participants in the lectures, especially David Godden, Fred Gifford, Todd Hedrick, Matt Ferkany, Laura Cabrera, Robyn Bluhm, Jamie Nelson, Matthew W. McKeon and Professor Peter Railton (who did me the honor of coming from Ann Arbor), and the students for their questions, comments, suggestions etc. and for our conversations over lunch and on many other occasions. Thanks also to Nicole Carolyn-Indira Shilling for inviting me to present my ideas at the MSU Philosophy Club. Many thanks especially to Professor Frederick Rauscher for organizing the lectures at MSU and for our ongoing philosophical discussions, not only on Kant's meta-ethics and the Kantian bioethical principle of respect for persons, but on some Rawlsian political issues too.

I would also like to thank some colleagues of the current research group I am working with, namely the *Global Consortium O3*: Our Brain, Our Selves, Our World (An International Research Consortium on Neuroscience, Ethics and Society.), coordinated by Professor Ilina Singh (Oxford University), especially those dealing with the neuroethics panels, namely Professors Julian Savulescu and Walter Sinnott-Armstrong for their comments to my "case-response" in our meeting at the Ashridge Business School (England, June 2016), supported by the Welcome Trust. I am also grateful for the opportunity to meet and to discuss some points with the North American neuroethicists, particularly Martha Farah and Steven Hyman. I was invited to be part of a thematic group in this consortium to contribute with my expertise in bioethics having done some research at The

Oxford Uehiro Centre for Practical Ethics. The ideas defended here of course do not represent the official view of the O3, but only my personal understanding of such matters.

INTRODUCTION

Reshaping the Field of Neuroethics

From time to time, a particular science achieves such great success that people are tempted to elevate it to the condition of *prima philosophia* and then to try to explain everything else from its perspective. Thus, physics becomes physicalism; history, historicism, and so on. Nowadays, the big science is the investigation of the nervous system, particularly *the brain*, as can be recognized by looking at the US B.R.A.I.N. Initiative (Brain Research through Advancing Innovative Neurotechnologies); the EU's Human Brain Project; Brazil's IINNT (a campus of the brain in Natal, RN), idealized by Miguel Nicolelis; the Institute of the Brain, which is also in Brazil (Porto Alegre, RS) and led by the Argentinian-born Ivan Izquierdo, etc. The main paradigm is, then, given by neuroscience and everything else seems to require its prefix: neurophilosophy, neuroeconomy, neuroeducation, neurotheology, neurolaw, neurotechnology, neuroethics, neuropolitics etc. I do not need to multiply examples to show that "neuromania" is upon us; that is, the belief that one needs to learn the workings of the brain to know anything at all. Thus, we seem to live in the age of "brainism" (Bakhurst, 2008). But what does it really mean to use "neuro" as a prefix to a word as it appears in the title of this book?

To answer this question and to clarify the main argument of this work, I would, in this introduction, like to present some of the general philosophical assumptions that guide my work both in bioethics and neuroethics and to propose reshaping the field of neuroethics towards what I here call "neurobioethics." My general argument can be put forward in this way:

1º–since the predominant use of "neuroethics" is ambiguous and may involve categorial and other errors in trying to extract normative implications directly from neuroscientific studies, the ethics of neuroscientific experiments must be based on classical bioethics despite the fact that we need also to overcome the intuitionist meta-ethical problems of the predominant normative theory using a new moral epistemology, namely *practical cognitivism*;

2º–now, despite the fact that classical bioethics is already well-armed with the main ethical guidelines to perform neuroscientific experiments on human beings in the right way, especially by applying the *prima facie* principle of respect for persons, it also needs some normative improvements towards a more unified account of *care* and *respect* since this unification can lead, for instance, to the concept of *caring respect*, which is crucial for a common and shareable morality in the public sphere;

3º–thus, by applying *practical cognitivism* and *caring respect* to the ethics of neuroscientific investigations and their associated neurotechologies, for example to the moral problems of cognitive enhancement using nootropics, we can better recognize that neuroethics is just a subfied of bioethics and not an independent branch of applied ethics; hence, *neurobioethics*.

Each of these steps in the argument will be made in the following three chapters; the first will be on the *meta-ethical* basis of neurobioethics, the second on the *normative* foundations of neurobioethics, and the last on some *practical* issues belonging to neurobioethics. In the end, the entire argument will reach the conclusion that we need to depart from neuroethics, unduly compromised with scientificism and utilitarianism, *towards neurobioethics*.

To explain in greater detail what neurobioethics is all about, I would first like to present some methodological remarks. In general, I will follow a Wittgensteinian orientation as given by the neurologist M. R. Bennett and the philosopher P. M. S. Hacker, who, in their excellent book *Philosophical Foundations of Neuroscience*, made clear what philosophy and neuroscience can do and what they cannot do: the former proceeds through *conceptual analyses*; the latter by doing *empirical investigations* (2003, 378f). Conceptual analysis is, then, in some sense *prior* and not reducible to empirical investigations (the sciences). Moreover, I will argue that Bennett and Hacker are right in holding that science must avoid being committed to metaphysical reductionism (2003, 355f). I will expand on this point soon.

Now, one remark I would like to make straight away is that the *neuroscience* of morality (sometimes used as one of the meanings of "neuroethics") is a worthy kind of investigation, but it cannot, by itself, provide a normative framework for dealing with research using humans as subjects. To accomplish that, we need (bio)*ethics*, which is an autonomous area of study. To think otherwise is to fall into scientificism; that is, into a metaphysics that leads to a partial and distorted understanding of reality. As Wittgenstein puts it (TLP, 6.52), we feel that even when all possible scientific questions have been answered, the problems of life remain untouched. Thus, the general aim of this section is to offer a broader picture of ethics as a *philosophical* enterprise in order to provide a background for the argument I will present and defend throughout this work.

I would, then, like to start with a clear definition of philosophy itself to make explicit what it can and cannot do, and to establish the foundations of neurobioethics. I take pure philosophy to be just *a search for wisdom*. In this sense, I would like to honor Potter's original bioethical project: "Mankind is urgently in need of new wisdom that will provide the 'knowledge of how to use knowledge' for man's survival and for improvement in the quality of life." (Potter 1971, 1) The author of the book *Bioethics, Bridge to the Future* goes on to clarify that the humanities and philosophy, understood as "love of wisdom," play an important role, together with the science of biology, in building the "science of survival" he calls "Bioethics." As can be seen, Potter emphasizes the two most important ingredients in achieving this new wisdom. Granted, philosophy is a search for wisdom, but what is *wisdom* after all?

I believe Potter was on the right track when he envisaged a kind of metaknowledge, namely *the knowledge of how* to use scientific knowledge for *ethical* purposes, rescuing in this way wisdom's *protagonist* role in our lives. That is to say, there are many different kinds of knowledge and philosophy cannot be conflated with any type: it is neither *common sense* nor *one of the natural or social sciences.* Philosophy is not common sense since it is not a-methodic and uncritical in the way common sense is, working through trial and error only; it is not full of unexamined beliefs or values; it is not "popular wisdom" either. On the contrary, philosophy is most critical of some conventional beliefs and practices.

Philosophy is not a particular natural science either since it does not proceed in experimental ways using empirical methods (induction, hypothetical-deductive, etc.) *to explain* causally natural phenomena, but rather works conceptually and argumentatively; it has no particular object, but everything is open to its reflection; it is *knowing-how to use scientific knowledge to improve the quality of our lives*. Nor is philosophy one of the social sciences since it does not attempt to understand or *to describe*, for instance, different moral traditions. Moreover, philosophy has, since classical times, been driven by ethical imperatives such as *Know thyself*! leading to the re-*cognition* of the limits of scientific knowledge itself. Thus, philosophy is non-naturalistic and its special status can be shown as follows: despite the fact that empirical sciences such as biology are the best way of explaining causally many facts concerning the world around us, science needs philosophy, both to refute radical skepticism –thus instituting the very possibility of scientific knowledge itself– and to establish ethical ends for its activities. The sciences cannot establish themselves in a circular way, that is, by asserting scientifically that there is scientific knowledge. To achieve this aim, we need a different kind of understanding, namely a philosophical one which shows that skepticism is nonsensical. Besides, both science and neurotechnology can be used to kill or to save lives, so it is paramount to ground them on a sound philosophy to ensure, to use Potter's words, man's survival and an improvement in quality of life, which is an *ethico-philosophical* end, not a scientific one.

It is also crucial to distinguish philosophy from the arts and the religions, especially from ideologies and other forms of sophistry. The arts and religions are *expressions* of human imagination. Religions are also based on non-cognitive grounds such as *dogma* and *faith* and feelings (e.g., fear and hope); on the contrary, philosophy cares for wisdom. Most religions postulate supranatural entities such as God, souls etc., while a sound philosophy cannot commit itself to such an ontology. An attempt to pass off a specific religion as scientific is an ideological one, as well as being an effort elevate science to metaphysical significance. An ideology is a set of beliefs and values that obscures part of reality; it disguises wishes and interests. Philosophy is above all committed to truth and to emancipation from false or hidden beliefs. It is not any sophist self-proclaimed possession of the ultimate truth, but a permanent search to improve wisdom. Besides, only philosophy is based on universal human values, whereas ideology and sophistry are based on specific ones.

A philosophy based on wisdom has an irreducible ethical component, and if the previous remarks are cogent, then it is easy to grasp the *autonomy* of ethics; namely, it is neither a science nor a religion. To conflate values (ethics) and facts (sciences) is to commit the naturalistic fallacy by defining non-natural concepts such as "good," "right" etc. in natural terms (e.g., more evolved). This is a category mistake which thus invalidates all conclusions. I will return to this point while discussing the problem of crisscrossing language-games (chapter 1).

Now, to avoid similar confusions, it is crucial to make the distinction between *ethics* and *morality*. Basically, I differentiate "ethics" as a philosophical discipline from "morality" as referring to particular value systems. First, then, I will sort out the main domain of philosophical ethics, and I will then provide a better definition of "morality" soon. Afterwards, I will construct a map of applied ethics to locate neurobioethics.

Ethics is normally seen as comprising three main spheres:

(i) Meta-ethics;
(ii) Normative Ethics and
(iii) Applied Ethics.

I will deal with each of these domains in the three chapters of this book, which sort out respectively the three main ideas of this work: one is meta-ethical (practical cognitivism as a substitute for the intuitionist basis of neurobioethics); another is normative (the concept of caring respect) and, finally, there is a practical one (the permissibility or not of cognitive enhancers) which is closely related to the three steps of the main argument as stated above.

Meta-ethics is, then, an examination of the epistemic and ontological status of ethics itself. For instance, some meta-ethical issues are whether moral knowledge exists (cognitivism *vs.* non-cognitivism); whether there are moral proprieties and whether they are natural ones (realism *vs.* anti-realism); whether morality is intrinsically motivating and so on. In chapter 1, I will develop the main tenets of a new moral epistemology to justify some meta-ethical and normative claims I make later, for instance, that one *knows-how* to respect a vulnerable subject of neuroscientific research (or not). Thus, I will argue that there is moral knowledge and that it is best understood as involving knowing-how to act, which goes under the label of "practical cognitivism" and will provide the meta-ethical grounds for neurobioethics.

Now, *normative ethics* deals with ways of distinguishing right from wrong, good from bad etc. in the moral sense. Normative ethics is currently divided into three main normative approaches: (i) *virtue ethics* (right is what a virtuous person would do in the circumstances); (ii) *consequentialism* (right is what brings the best results) and (iii) *deontology* (right actions may have worth in themselves and be prescribed by universal norms). In chapter 2, I will try to show that there is a way of overcoming this tripartite division, making, for instance, an ethics of care and an ethics of universal respect compatible and congruent, thus leading to attitudes such as *caring respect* which may have important applications in all domains of life, including in neurobioethics.

Applied ethics is the practical domain where particular moral issues are analyzed using a normative approach, for instance, bioethical problems such as whether voluntary euthanasia is permissible; neuroethical problems such as whether cognitive enhancement by pharmaceutical means is morally acceptable for teenagers; roboethical issues such as whether artificial agents have rights; ecoethical issues such as whether biodiversity has intrinsic worth; zooethical issues such as whether non-human animals can be used in neuroscientific experiments; etc. In chapter 3, I will discuss neuroethical problems in great detail, especially cognitive enhancement. As can be seen, there are apparently many subfields within applied ethics: bioethics, neuroethics, roboethics, ecoethics, zooethics, etc., which deal with practical, day-to-day moral problems using *normative* approaches grounded on *meta-ethics*. I will better clarify the interconnections between these subfields of applied ethics below, explaining why we need to walk in the direction of neurobioethics.

From a philosophical point of view, meta-ethical problems have priority. That is to say, a philosopher must first make sure that the meta-ethical bases are well settled in order to find the best normative account to address practical concerns. It is almost unnecessary to say that applied ethics has priority in our everyday lives. I will deal with some practical problems in this book, especially issues surrounding the use of drugs for cognitive enhancement as well as treatment to illustrate the meta-ethical and normative points I propose here.

Having made these distinctions of the main domains of ethics, it is now possible to better distinguish it from *morality*. Consider Roger Crisp's definition of a morality (2006, 9):

> … a set of cognitive and conative states, including beliefs, desires, and feelings, which leads its possessors among other things to (*a*) view certain actions as wrong (that is, morally forbidden), and hence to be avoided, (*b*) feel guilt and/or shame as a result of performing such actions, and (*c*) blame others who perform such actions.

Thus, a particular morality can be understood as a value system, that is, a set of beliefs, practices, norms, virtues, feelings, etc., which lead us to regard particular actions as right or wrong. In this sense, there seem to be many value systems: Christian morality; liberal morality; Buddhist morality; communist morality etc. Whether this plurality of value systems implies relativism is an open question, as it is whether there are sufficient *shared values* to postulate "*the* common morality". I will discuss this point in chapter 2.

Now, it seems clear that we have to accept the plurality of value systems, and not only as a matter of fact. If the definition of philosophy as a search for wisdom is sound, and if wisdom has to do with the re-cognition of the limits of knowledge, then we are bound to accept *agnosticism* in metaphysics and its pluralist implications as a matter of principle. That is to say, specific moral systems may be based on *antagonic* metaphysical assumptions. For instance, one moral system may contain religious beliefs, while others can be built on naturalist values. Moral systems express, then, different worldviews, but we can only sketch a *finite* ontology. This finite ontology, though, may have important ethical purposes anyway. Thus, we may take a *methodological* naturalist approach to moral phenomena, but we cannot assume *metaphysical* naturalism in a reductivistic or eliminationistic manner. This philosophical point has important practical consequences for what the sciences, for example neuroscience, can do to help us to understand morality. As we will see in this work, reshaping neuroethics in the direction of neurobioethics prevents us from committing a naturalistic fallacy and avoids many other problems.

Even if some degree of value pluralism should be accepted, not only as a matter of fact, but also in principle, it does not follow that radical moral relativism is true or that moral skepticism should be subscribed as a consequence. Normative relativism cannot be conflated with descriptive relativism. It is a *category mistake* to identify normative claims with matters of fact; that is, to try to infer an *ought* (a prescriptive statement) directly from an *is* (a descriptive proposition). From the idea that philosophy is a search for wisdom, we may extract the project of building up *a* common and sharable morality (henceforth, *a* CS-Morality) to make value pluralism reasonable. To rephrase the American political philosopher John Rawls (1993, xvii), there is no "the fact of a plurality of reasonable but incompatible comprehensive doctrines," but rather *pluralism must be made reasonable* through *a* CS-Morality. Such *a* moral system is the *sine qua non* condition for the pacific co-existence of and cooperation among divergent value systems. Therefore, reasonable value pluralism is only possible under the assumption of *a* CS-Morality. Radical ethical relativism turns out, then, to be false.

A similar argument can be presented to reject moral skepticism. As we saw above, there are many kinds of knowledge, and the denial of knowing-how, which presupposes the acquired capacity to follow norms, is simply self-contradictory. Actually, we can show that the skeptic presupposes what he wants to deny. This argument opens the door to constructing a moral epistemology based on the idea that there is moral knowledge and that it is best understood as involving knowing-how. This is the main purpose of chapter 1: to present the meta-ethical basis of neurobioethics and open the door to establishing a normative ethical theory. To illustrate, a person may know-how *to respect* other person, who happen to be a vulnerable being, namely in a *caring* way (or not). Once again, this meta-ethical claim leads us to the normative idea of *a* CS-Morality based on, as we will see in greater detail in chapter 2, *mutual care* and *reciprocal respect*.

I would now like to examine some interconnections between the subfields of *applied ethics*, especially the links between bioethics and neuroethics, and to present the domain of neurobioethics. I started this introduction by identifying Potter's project of bioethics as a bridge between the empirical sciences and the humanities to achieve a *new wisdom* that leads to an improvement in quality of life. Unfortunately, this is not the predominant use of the word "bioethics" nowadays. In fact, its main employment relates to the principles and values of biomedicine and other health sciences only. As can be seen clearly, this is not what the very same Potter years ago called "global bioethics" in his later book, which includes many environmental issues and is built on Leopold's legacy, namely on the project of an ethics of land. Too bad for us that this is also not the main use of "global bioethics," since most bioethicists use it to refer to international bioethical issues. Thus, I would like to distinguish three main uses of "bioethics", referring to: (i) holist bioethics; (ii) special bioethics and (iii) global bioethics. We should bear in mind, however, that a truly *philosophical bioethics*, guided by the conception of philosophy spelled out above, maintains interconnections among all these domains.

How can we distinguish holist from special bioethics? I think that one way of seeing the differences is to refer to Potter's original project but to rename it *holistic bioethics* in the sense that it includes a moral concern for the environment and non-human animals too; that is, it *cares for life as a whole*. This fits well with what Fritz Jahr, perhaps the first person to have used the term "bioethics", had in mind when he proposed the following principle: "Respect every living being on principle as an end in itself and treat it, if possible, as such." (Jahr 2012, 4) Of course, there is the issue of whether we should respect every single living being or, as Leopold held, we should rather revere the biotic community as a whole. Leopold's ethical principle was, in his famous *A Sand County Almanac*, sorted out in these terms: "A thing is right when it tends to preserve the integrity, stability, and beauty of the biotic community. It is wrong when it tends otherwise." (1993, 16) The implications of these principles, namely Jahr's and Leopold's criteria to distinguish right from wrong actions, may lead to different practices. To illustrate: the former seems to lead necessarily to vegetarianism or even to veganism; the latter, not necessarily. Unfortunately, I cannot pursue this issue here, but I would like to emphasize that *holist bioethics* would then amount to a general attitude of respect for life as a whole including the environment and non-human animals.

Now, *special bioethics,* in contrast, may refer exclusively to the principles and values needed to carry out scientific experiments that use human beings as subjects in the health sciences. It relates mainly but not exclusively to biomedical experiments. In fact, the classical "bioethical" book *Principles of Biomedical Ethics* starts by identifying them in its very first sentence: "Biomedical ethics, or bioethics, …" (Beauchamp & Childress 2013, vii). This identification is, however, misleading since it seems clear that there are deep interconnections between human well-being and a healthy environment. Moreover, an anthropologist does not do research *on* human beings, but *with* human subjects. Unfortunately, this is still the predominant use, which gives us a very limited understanding of bioethics in general. Now, sub-fields of special bioethics include *clinical* bioethics, *neonatal* bioethics, etc. and arguably, *neuro*-bioethics itself. As we will see, neurobioethics is a subfield of special bioethics. Since I will, for didactic reasons, focus on *special bioethics* throughout this book, I will return to this point later to complement this exposition.

In addition, there is *global bioethics*, which deals with bioethical issues within international relations between countries. This is, for instance, what is mainly established in domestic or regional bioethical treaties, for instance, the Oviedo Convention, which prescribes norms for the European Community on many bioethical issues. With this in mind, we Americans should, perhaps, have an Interamerican Bioethics Declaration as we have for Human Rights (San José, 1969). There is, of course, The UNESCO Universal Declaration on Bioethics and Human Rights, but still, it seems justifiable to consider what is specific for the Americas as a distinct region. Now, some bioethicists are skeptical about whether we can reach a global consensus on such questions (e.g., Engelhardt 2006). In this work, I will briefly compare the North American and the Brazilian ways of doing bioethics (and neuroethics) in order to make sense of the idea of *a* CS-Morality, but I will not, for reasons of space, discuss all the issues related to global bioethics.

To avoid confusion and misunderstandings, we must keep in mind that all these distinctions are useful to the extent that they help us to focus on particular neurobioethical issues, but that they should not make us lose sight of the forest. Thus, I have proposed using the expression "philosophical bioethics" to maintain the idea that *wisdom* must guide our actions in all these domains and to synthetize the results of particular subdomains into a comprehensive understanding of our moral lives. For instance, it could guide us in discussing neurobioethical issues such as whether we should allow smart drugs to be used in high schools and universities not only for treatment, but also as enhancers.

Before proposing a map to guide us through the landscape of neurobioethics, I would like to clarify better the uses of the neologism "neuroethics." It has, following Roskies' 2002 famous distinction (see references), become commonplace to distinguish two main meanings of "neuroethics", either to refer to: (i) the ethics needed to conduct neuroscientific research and its technological applications (briefly, neuro*ethics*) or (ii) the neuroscientific studies of ethics or, better, morality (briefly, *neuro*ethics). To illustrate, I would like to mention the way the *Global Consortium O3*, in its first meeting, organized the main panels:

1° – Ethics of neuroscience (Chaired by Professor Julian Savulescu, Oxford University);

2° – Neuroscience of ethics (Chaired by Professor Walter Sinnott-Armstrong, Duke University).

In chapter 1 of this book, I will present a case relating to cognitive enhancers and some of the questions on this topic we discussed in the first panel using neurobio*ethics* as the ethics needed for neuroscientific research and some of its neurotechnological applications.

Since I will, in this work, focus on the first group of issues, that is, on the *ethics of neuroscience*, I would here like to mention the main questions the first panel aims to investigate over the next couple of years: (i) the challenges of neurotechnology (e.g., the use of machines to read the human mind, brain–computer interfaces etc.); (ii) the possibility of predicting behavior and controlling individuals (e.g., the use of neurostimulation through tDCS, TMS and DBS); iii) issues surrounding the use of automated systems, especially apps, to increase well-being (e.g., the use of virtual reality to treat mental disorders), etc. I will examine these issues in detail in chapter 3 (cf. www.o3brain.org for further information).

The ethical significance of neuroscientific investigations using human beings as subjects of research or their potential applications is evident. For instance, in the first group, there are conflicts between the increasing accuracy of mind-reading machines against the right to *mental* privacy; in the second, the potential therapeutic benefits of new procedures to treat mental disorders, but, at the same time, the unknown long term effects of, for instance, the use of mood (e.g., lithium) or cognitive enhancers (e.g., amphetamine, commercially known as Adderall®) and issues related to individual identity *and personhood*; in the third, the conflicts between increasing efficacy *versus* potential abuses of technological devices.

Considering these issues, the first panel of the O3 group sorted out some key research problems:

1) How would the development of more powerful neuroimaging that was better equipped to detect consciousness affect the ethics of end-of-life medical decisions?
2) How should decisions to deploy medical interventions which directly affect the human mind be made?
3) Such interventions raise questions about what role, if any, they should have in the criminal justice system, and whether their use would unacceptably threaten human freedom?

4) How is 'care' constituted when it is delivered via an algorithm, or a robot? Are there particular concerns about care delivery in the context of mental health and well-being?
5) How should mental health and well-being apps be regulated?
6) Is there a universal morality that should guide normative judgments about interventions to improve moral behavior and decision-making?

I will give a brief response, with no intention of presenting a final answer, to some of these questions in chapters 1 and 2. In general though, in this book, I will focus more on issues around the ethics of neuroscience. To be even more specific, I will investigate the permissibility of one special kind of *enhancement*, namely the improvement of cognitive capabilities either using conventional (education) or nor-conventional (genetic or pharmacological) means. This issue relates to questions 1, 4 and 5. To deal adequately with neuroenhancement, I will defend *a* CS-Morality comprising care and respect, which are based on practical cognitivism, to respond to question 6 and, to some extent, questions 2 and 3.

Now, the other meaning of "*neuro*ethics", namely the *neuroscience of ethics*, which would perhaps be better referred to as "the neuroscientific studies of moral phenomena" is a very recent topic of research. According to the opening speech by Professor Walter Sinnott-Armstrong in the above mentioned O3 first meeting, "since the first fMRI study of ethics in Brazil in 2001, neuroscientists have published an increasing number of sophisticated experiments on various aspects of moral judgments, decisions, and emotions." (http://o3brain.org/about-o3/). Actually, as far as I know, the first Brazilian fMRI study on the neural correlates of moral judgement was published in *Neurology* (Oliveira-Souza & Moll, 2000) and predates the first neuroethics studies by Joshua Greene (2001). In any case, the works of the Brazilian neuroscientist Jorge Moll, from the IDOR (Instituto D'Or Pesquisa e Ensino, RJ) are certainly pioneering in the field of the neuroscience of moral judgement, as Professor Sinnott-Armstrong correctly pointed out. Now, the neuroscience of morality deals with questions such as whether there is free will, the role of reason and emotions in moral decision-making etc. There is even some hope that neuroscience can help to settle *normative* issues, for instance, whether a deontological approach or a consequentialist one must be assumed in dealing with moral issues regarding what to do. To give an example: recently, Joshua Greene (2013, 289f; 2017,11) was still trying to make the point that neuroscience leads to utilitarianism as "the *ultimate standard*" against which to judge our moral thinking, contrary to deontology or virtue ethics.

I am somewhat skeptical about whether *neuro*ethics can deliver on most of its ambitious promises. In fact, I think that it is even an inappropriate expression since the neuroscience of morality still is just *science*, not *ethics*. It is a descriptive enterprise, not a normative one. That is to say, strictly speaking a neuro-*scientific* study of morality is scientific only: it presupposes *explanations* of what is going on in our brain when we think about moral issues, but it cannot *prescribe* a particular moral way of thinking about them and acting accordingly. This is one of the main reasons why we need to move in the direction of neuro*bioethics*.

I would then argue for this thesis, namely that the use of "*neuro*ethics" as a neuroscientific study of ethics commits a category mistake by crisscrossing, so to speak, two different language-games (descriptive and normative), and, consequently, it misuses the concepts "neuro" and "ethics." If this is right, then there is only one employment of "neuroethics" that makes sense, namely, an examination of the ethics of neuroscientific studies and their neurotechnological applications (neuro*ethics*). Therefore, we should stick to what was perhaps one of the first definitions of "neuroethics" given by William Safire at the San Francisco inaugural meeting *Neuroethics: Mapping the Field*, back in 2002: "*the examination of what is right and wrong, good and bad about the treatment of, perfection of, or unwelcome invasion of and worrisome manipulation of the human brain*." (https://danablog.org). I believe this is one of the best definitions of "neuroethics" put forward up to now, and it reveals clear interconnections with traditional bioethics.

Suppose, however, one disagrees with my claim and would like to insist on using the word "neuroethics" in such a way that includes the neuroscientific studies of morality. Well, I will not fight over words or labels here, but I would rather ask why we should attribute any special status to neuroscience anyway. After all, a neuroimage of the brain activity is insufficient to determine whether we should allow, for instance, active, nonvoluntary euthanasia. Besides, I would object that a *scientific* study of morality is certainly relevant, but then I would invite my adversary to think of whether ethnology (or anthropology), sociobiology, primatology, etc. are not as crucial as neuroscience. We cannot certainly hope to use fMRI to look for particular rights or obligations in our brains since they are historical and social constructions, even if they are justified using natural laws. Furthermore, neuroethicists are making an interesting move these days to overcome a unilateral approach, namely they are looking at society as a whole to better understand what is going on in our brains when we make moral decisions. For these reasons, I would stand by the single use of "neuro*ethics*" as the ethics of neuroscience. This is, at least, the main use in this work of "neuro*ethics*", and I will present further arguments later for rehaping it as neuro*bio*ethics.

This restriction brings us to the task of deepening the analysis of the interfaces between neuroethics so conceived, and bioethics. I would then like to quote here the predominant view on this point given by one of the participants of the O3, namely the psychologist Marta J. Farah: "New ethical issues are arising as neuroscience gives us unprecedented ways to understand *the human mind and to predict, influence, and even control it*. These issues lead us beyond the boundaries of bioethics into the philosophy of mind, psychology, theology, law and neuroscience itself. It is this larger set of issues that has…earned it a name of its own." (Farah 2010, 2; italics added) There are two main ideas here: one is the need for interdisciplinarity; the other, the idea that neuroscientific knowledge leads to new technological applications and, consequently, gives us ways to manipulate the brain to control the mind. The first point is common to many studies, including bioethics. However, the second issue just reveals that the proper domain of neuroethics is *the ethics of neuroscience* and its neurotechnological applications. Therefore, to the extent that neuroethicists deal with questions on mental disorders (panic, anxiety, depression, psychosis, schizophrenia etc.), physical brain impairments or addiction, autism, neuroenhancement or treatment, etc. in *scientific research* or *clinical* practices, they seem to fall into the traditional domain of bioethics.

Once again, perhaps the critic could easily respond to the question *How is neuroethics different from bioethics?* in terms of neuroexceptionalism (Illes 2017, ix). That is to say, unlike other organs, the brain connects each of us to who we are; that is, the brain is very special because it links us to our identity and it is the organ of human mind. There are many interesting facts about our brain, but does it pose a new normative or evaluative challenge? No doubt, it has a very special role, for instance, in our capacity to make decisions, in our autonomy, and so on. But the *ethical* question is: should we respect autonomous decisions? Then, it does not follow that it makes sense, as we will see, to speak in terms of "the moral brain." The person, not one of her organs, is the moral entity to be respected. Rightly, Bennett and Hacker (2003, p.68) called this mistake a "mereological fallacy." In other words, mereological fallacies (taking *parts* such as our brains as if they were the *whole* of an organic being) have no place in a sound neurobioethics; that is, we must know-how to *respect persons* as whole biopsychosocial entities, not only their nervous systems or their brains.

Is there really something distinctive to the ethics of neuroscience which justifies the use of "a new name for a new field?" According to Steven E. Hyman, "The major justification for demarcating neuroethics from the broader field of bioethics derives from the special status of the brain (Roskies, 2002), which is the causal underpinning of our conscious mental lives and of our behavior." (2013, 96). Once again, however, it does look reductionist to consider only the brain: even if it is special for many reasons (billions of neurons making trillhons of neural connections), it seems that we should regard the human being as a whole, as a unity. We must avoid what Bakhurst (2008, 415) calls "brainism," or the view (i) that an individual's mental life is constituted by states, events and processes in her brain, and (ii) that psychological attributes may legitimately be ascribed to the brain only. We must rather consider the person, not the brain, as a whole in relation to nature and society. Granted, controlling the brain is one way of controlling the mind, but this is not the whole story. If it were, neuroethics would be justified because neuroscience really has given us unprecedented ways "to predict, influence, and even to control [the mind]". (Farah 2010, 2). This may well be so, but the real ethical question is under what conditions this power is justified? My quick answer is this: if we are dealing with mental disorders in an experimental setting, then it seems clear that, for instance in the US, the Belmont principles (respect for persons, beneficence and justice) fully apply; if we are discussing other issues, for instance, around the political control of another's mind, then there are legitime or illegitimate ways of doing it, but caring and respecting persons seems always to be morally required. That is to say, respecting persons entails not manipulating their minds, especially if they are part of vulnerable populations, for instance, prisoners or individuals with mental disorders. I will return to the issues of mental disorders in the last chapter, but it seems clear that caring respect requires working to increasea person's autonomy, not enslaving her.

Bearing all these points in mind, I can, finally, sort out the main interconnections between bioethics and neuroethics and arrive at the proper domain of what I have called "neurobio*ethics.*" Actually, there is already a vague use of this expression since it seems clear that some scientific developments in neuroscience raise bioethical questions. Concerns in the area of neurobioethics are put in these terms:

> Some of these debates include whether particular interventions represent treatment or enhancement, the use or misuse of neurogenetic and neuroimaging data, moral ambiguities surrounding the use of neural allo- and xenotransplantation, and ethical dilemmas arising within the contexts of neuroscientific policy, clinical practice and the scope and tenor of current and future research directions.
> (http://www.unescobiochair.org/neurobioethics/).

As can be seen, neurobioethics does not rely exclusively on the neuroscience of ethics. It also incorporates the social dimensions of doing research on human beings as, for instance, the details of the infamous Tukesggee case remind us. Granted, neuroscience poses new ethical challenges, but the main issue at stake is how we can deal with them and neurobioethics has the right normative framework, for instance, the principle respect for persons.

It is also worth remembering that the *National Commission for the Protection of Human Subjects of Biomedical and Behavioral Research*, the publisher of the Belmont Report which sorted out the principle of respect for *persons,* was very interdisciplinary. Another difference, then, between *neuro*ehtics (driven by neuroscientific investigations of the moral brain) and neurobio*ethics* is that the latter is more interdisciplinary. It encompasses contributions from moral psychology, anthropology, ethnology, sociology, etc. *and* society, while tradional neuroethics is limited to *one* science alone: the neuroscience of morality.

Another huge difference is that neurobioethics does not make inadaquete conceptual and factual transpositions from the neuroscientific investigations directly into ethics. For instance, it may well be a neuroscientific "conclusion" that personhood is an illusion rooted in the brain (Farah and Heberlein 2010, p.321), but it does not follow that persons do not exist or that this concept cannot be constructed from a more interdisciplinary perspective, namely from a social and juridical stance. I will return to this point later when presenting an argument against Farah's conclusion. For these and other reasons, it is better to work with neurobioethics and not with traditional neuroethics. Consequently, one of the most fundamental questions I would like to ask in this book is whether or not special bioethics is normatively well equipped to treat all the new ethical challenges posed by neuroscience.

Whether neuroethics is just part of bioethics is, then, not a new debate. Some thinkers hold that it is not, while others maintain that these problems can indeed be dealt with within the traditional bioethical framework, for instance by using the basic norms of the *Belmont Report* (especially respect for persons, a concept some neuroethicists think is an illusion), which will be commented on later, or some variant of these such as principlism, autonomism, etc. The Belmont normative framework may be sufficient to cope with the challenges presented by neuroscience and neurotechnology, and if this is the case, as I believe it is, and there are no other neuroethical issues left out, then neuro*ethics* (in the sense of an"ethics of neuroscience") turns out to be just a subfield of bioethics: *neurobioethics*.

The main normative problem this work addresses is consequently as follows: which are the basic norms needed to deal with the ethical challenges arising from neuroscience and neurotechnology? Thus, another thesis I will argue for is this one: while we are doing neuroscientific research, neuroexperiments and applying neurotechnologies using human subjects, the bioethical normative framework works well, but we need also to get the right one. That is to say, in chapter 2 I will support the *The Belmont Guidelines*, and criticize other normative approaches derived from them such as principlism, autonomism, etc. I will also in this chapter criticize the main attempts of some neuroethicists, such as Greene and Farah, to establish utilitarianism as the normative ethics for dealing with the problems of the ethics of neuroscience. Thus, I will, after correcting the metaethical problems of bioethics in chapter 1, find a way of integrating care and respect into an unified normative approach. Consequently, I will use the expression "neurobioethics" to refer to a particular sub-field of bioethics assuming the *onus probandi* that this hypothesis can be demonstrated; that is, that traditional bioethicists got the moral principles of this domain right. That is to say, well-understood (neuro)bioethics has the necessary normative resources to deal with the main ethical challenges neuroscience and neurotechnology have presented so far. What is further needed is just willingness to follow principles such as respect for persons in our caring practices and scientific research. Briefly, what is needed is *knowing-how to respect neuroscientific subjects*, namely in a caring way. This is one of the main ideas of this work and is presented under the label "neurobioethics."

This last point reveals also the main justification for this book. I would like to put it in this way: in her excellent work "Neuroscience and Neuroethics in the 21th Century", the psychologist Martha J. Fahar (2013, 761) reviews the main neuroscientific challenges facing us nowadays, especially the enhancement of mental functioning, neuroscience-based education, neuromarketing, the new roles of criminal justice and the law, etc. and presents three new ones: (i) neuroliteracy for the neurocentury, (ii) ownership and control of neurotechnology and (iii) avoiding nihilism. The spirit of this book can then be seen as a response to the third "new" challenge: how can we prevent neuroscience's physicalist explanations of human behavior lapsing into nihilism? My view, then, is that persons are *not* mere physical objects and must be respected in a caring manner as moral entities while we are doing applied ethics, especially neurobioethics. This will be illustrated in chapter 3 when I discuss the permissibility of cognitive enhancement. In fact, I will present an argument to refute the idea that personhood is just an illusion. This will make it possible to work with the principle of respect for persons, to defend a person-centered healthcare system, to put the person before the patient or the subject of neuroscientific research or the use of neurotechnologies, etc. To accomplish this goal, my main proposal is to redirect neuroethics, freeing it from its naturalistic and utilitarian assumptions, towards neurobio*ethics*.

CHAPTER 1

META-ETHICS: THE EPISTEMIC FOUNDATIONS OF NEUROBIOETHICS

I would like to start this work by stating its general aim, namely to sort out the field of neurobioethics and ground its meta-ethical and normative assumptions. To achieve this goal, I will in this first chapter present a meta-ethical theory, particularly a new moral epistemology, I call "practical cognitivism." I propose this as a substitute for the intuitionist assumptions of the predominant normative ethical theory in bioethics, namely, the so-called "four principles approach" or "principlism" as presented in the classical book *Principles of Biomedical Ethics* (Beauchamp & Childress, 2013). This normative view is, as perhaps it is well-known, based on the *prima facie* norms of (i) respect for autonomy (*one ought to respect the autonomous choices of subjects of scientific research/patients*); (ii) non-maleficence (*one ought to refrain from inflicting harm*); (iii) beneficence (*one ought to do good and prevent or remove harm*) and (vi) justice (*one ought to treat people fairly*). The principles will be better explained soon as well as the meta-ethical foundations. Now, the basic idea of practical cognitivism is that moral knowledge involves knowing-how, for instance, to take care of a vulnerable being or respect a person, not only in the technical sense, but in the moral one too.

Before presenting this new epistemology to ground caring practices in neurobioethics, I will, in the first section of this chapter, explore some interconnections between bioethics and neuroethics and look for their interfaces in dealing with particular moral cases. In the second section, I will identify the main problem with the predominant theory; that is, it leads to irresoluble moral dilemmas, which is enough in itself to propose better normative foundations for neurobioethics. In the third section, then, I will present the main tenets of practical cognitivism and start to explore its normative connections, for instance, by asking under which conditions we may say that a person *knows-how* to respect a person *in a caring manner*.

Following that, in the next two chapters, I will extract the normative and practical implications of practical cognitivism. In the second chapter "Normative Ethics: Integrating Care and Respect" I will present a way of overcoming some divergences in normative theory especially between, on the one hand, care ethicists and, on the other hand, those working with respect for universal rights and justice, looking for a way to integrate them into a single concept, that is, caring respect. This will allow me to ground neurobioethics *normatively*. It seems clear that we must take care of all aspects of vulnerable individuals (including the brain) as well as respect a person's right to self-determination. The internal connection between caring and respecting, however, is not clear at all, and that is why I will present the concept of *caring respect* as referring to a fundamental attitude in neurobioethics. In the last chapter, "Caring Respect in Neurobioethics," I will *apply* the normative results to some neurobioethical issues, focusing on cognitive enhancement, as a way of testing both the new epistemology and the concept of caring respect.

1.1 – Interfaces between bioethics and neuroethics

To begin with, I would like to present a case which I am going to use to illustrate the meta-ethical points in this chapter and the practical ones throughout the rest of the book. I have, in my previous works, analyzed three *neonatal* bioethical cases (one in the US, one in Brazil and one in the UK).[1] Here, however, I will present one of the cases the O3 group analyzed in the first panel of its first meeting, chaired by Professor Julian Savulescu (Oxford University), having as respondents Steve Hyman, Debra Mathews and me, and the researchers Hannah Maslen and Jonathan Pugh. One of the hypothetical cases put forward to exemplify some problems with the ethics of neuroscience was phrased in these terms:

> Aysha is 16 and attends a school in a poor section of town. The school is an example of the general state of state funded schools in the country; it is overcrowded, the students are underperforming and unmotivated, and the teachers don't have sufficient training or time to support high educational achievement. The regional governing body for education has initiated a novel plan to support higher achievement in all state-funded secondary

[1] For more details: Dall'Agnol, D. *Care and Respect in Bioethics* (Newcastle: Cambridge Scholars, 2016), 7f. In that book, I discussed the cases from the perspective of *respectful care*. For a critical comment on my book see: Azevedo & Andrade, 2019. Here I will construct the concept of *caring respect*, but, as we will see in the next chapter, they may turn out to be two sides of the same coin.

> schools, by offering free cognitive enhancing drugs to both students and teachers. The state will also offer additional training days for teachers, and reward incentives for students who achieve certain goals. These benefits are open to all, regardless of whether they choose to accept the drugs or not. The decision to accept cognitive enhancing drugs is initially made by the school, and, if the school decides to accept, then individuals and families will opt in or opt out of the programme.[2]

This is a hypothetical case (which obviously could be a real one in countries such as Brazil and, perhaps, even in many cities across the US and UK), but it illustrates a series of moral issues in the interfaces between bioethics and neuroethics.[3] The case raises several ethical questions related to cognitive enhancers that will be dealt in chapter 3, but I would simply like to ask at this point: could we say that such an experimental program, as proposed in the Aysha case, shows real caring respect for the juvenile students themselves? To answer this *ethical* question, I will first propose practical cognitivism tied to a first principle of ethics to revise what each middle level norm of the predominant bioethical approach requires and, second, apply in a more detailed way the concept of caring respect to the case at hand.

Now, if we ask "under which conditions would respect really be caring?" in this case, as in any case indeed, we, surprisingly, will find out that in fact *we do not know*! This is an epistemic failure and that is why we need first of all to rethink the meta-ethical and normative basis of (neuro)bioethics. To illustrate this point, I would like to present two pieces of evidence. First, as John Lantos and William Meadow argued (2006), neonatology has gone through 3 distinct phases: (i) the era of innovation and individualism (1965-1982): this was the era of the technological imperative: if something *can* be done to save a premature baby, it *must* be done; (ii) the era of exposed ignorance (1982-1992) doctors *did not know how* to apply Baby Doe guidelines (my emphasis); (iii) the end of progress (1992 …): doctors/researchers simply ask parents what they really want. Several points call our attention in this brief history of neonatology: first, the lack of a particular kind of knowledge, namely *knowing-how*, which may well be one reason for malpractice, negligence, etc.; second, giving patients or subjects of scientific experiments whatever they want seems

---

[2] This case and the questions raised to respond can be found here: http://o3brain.org/2016/10/12/panel-one-ethics-of-neuroscience/

[3] At this point, it is interesting to note that both the neologisms "bioethics" and "neuroethics" had a very similar use back at the beginning of the 1970's. For instance, in his paper "Neuro-ethics of 'Waking' in the Newborn" (*Percept Mot Skills*, 1973; 37: 235-245), Pontius was already referring to the overlooked moral questions of biomedical ethics in the context of basic and clinical neuroscience.

unrealistic and may also lead to unethical outcomes. Here we realize also that we need to rethink the normative basis of bioethics, especially the status of the principle of respect for autonomy. Therefore, it looks like we still live in an era of moral ignorance.

This seems then to be the best place to point out that neuroscience can actually help us to understand better *the facts* of the case. As it is perhaps well known, magnetic resonance (MR) technology has revolutionized imaging of the brain. It can provide detailed images of the cerebrum, cerebellum, etc., helping not only more accurately to diagnose severe impairments by identifying specific areas of brain damage, but also to study the normal or abnormal development of a person's brain capacities. Now, one of the concerns of the consortium O3 is to understand how the development of more powerful neuro-imaging, better equipped to detect consciousness, would, just to illustrate, affect the ethics of end-of-life medical decisions.[4] The famous Terri Schiavo case is a good example of how more sophisticated neuroimaging technology could have helped to decide whether to withdraw life-sustaining treatment or not. Neuroimaging can support the prediction of future neurological outcomes; that is, it can *instrumentally* help to establish the degree and type of future disabilities given such and such brain injuries (e.g., serious motor, learning or sensory impairments, etc.).[5] However, whether we should withhold or withdraw life-sustaining treatment is an *ethical* question, which cannot be purely decided through neuroimaging. Now, the point to be investigated is whether Aysha has some cognitive impairment and needs treatment. Moreover, is she a person capable of autonomous decisions? In which way neuroscience can help to answer these questions? I will return to this point later.

---

[4] As I explained in the introduction of the present book, this is one of the questions I would like to address here. Question 1 was: "How would the development of more powerful neuro-imaging that was better equipped to detect consciousness affect the ethics of end-of-life medical decisions?" For instance, in the case of Shiavo, a brain-damaged woman in a persistent vegetative state for many years, it seems clear that neuroscience could help in explaining her "behaviors" as emerging from a decorticate brain, without cognition or consciousness. For further information on this case see: Caplan, A. *et al.* (eds) *The Case of Terri Schiavo* (New York: Prometheus Books, 2006), p. 133.

[5] For an interesting proposal of how to deal with this problem in premature babies see: Wilkinson, D. *Death or Disability*? The 'Carmentis Machine' and decision-making for critically ill children. (Oxford: Oxford University Press, 2013). I believe, however, that Wilkinson gives too much weight to autonomy, so it has, as we will see in chapter 2, the same problems as Engelhardt's autonomist views does, namely it may lead to *uncaring* respect.

The second piece of evidence relates to caring practices: we seem not to know also the proper objects of care and respect and the attitudes they require. That is to say, in philosophical ethics, we are in no better position than neonatologists were (and perhaps still are) in the era of exposed ignorance. Consider, for example's sake, Nel Nodding's analysis of care (2013, 69): "logically, we have the following situation (W, X) is a caring relation if and only if: (i) W cares for X (as described in the one-caring: sympathy, intrinsic valuation ...) and (ii) X recognizes that W cares for X." Nodding's conceptual analysis (spelling out the necessary and sufficient conditions for applying "care") is *circular* (the *analysandum* "care" cannot figure in the *analysans*) and even presents *non-necessary* conditions (the cared-for, for instance Terri Schiavo, does not need to recognize the one-caring. Therefore, the conditions conjointly are not sufficient. That is why we still need to engage in a serious philosophical task, that is, re-analyze fundamental concepts such as "care," "respect," etc.[6]

How did we come to such a state of not knowing-how to care or respect in a proper way? This is not, obviously, the place to reconstruct the entire history of bioethics, but a few brief remarks on the development of this field of applied ethics will help us to understand better the need for a *new moral epistemology* capable of showing us how to respect in a caring manner. What we could today call "special bioethics," to distinguish it from *global* (in Potter's sense)[7] or *holistic* bioethical approaches (in Jahr's sense),[8] deals exclusively with scientific experiments for therapeutic purposes

---

[6] It is worth recalling here that, on this methodological point, most bioethicists agree that one of the main contributions philosophers can make is to analyze concepts. According to Daniel Callahan, director of the prestigious Hastings Center, there are three main tasks for bioethicists: "definition of issues, methodological strategies, and procedures for decision-making." (Callahan 2007, p.19) See also chapter 3 entitled "The Philosophers: Clarifying the Concepts" of the book *The Birth of Bioethics* (Jonsen 1998).

[7] Until recently, the American physician Van Rensselaer Potter was believed to have coined the neologism "bioethics" to refer to a science of survival forged in these terms: "A science of survival must be more than science alone, and I therefore propose the term *Bioethics* in order to emphasize the two most important ingredients in achieving the new wisdom that is so desperately needed: biological knowledge and human values." (Potter 1971, 1) In his later work, Potter referred to his concern of life as a whole in terms of a "global bioethics," which builds on Leopold's Land Ethics (cf. Potter, V. R. *Global Bioethics*. East Lansing: MSU Press, 1988).

[8] Actually, the German Theologian Fritz Jahr is now believed to have coined the word "bioethics" back in 1927, subsuming his general moral concerns under a single principle: "Respect every living being on principle as an end in itself and treat it, if possible, as such." (Jahr 2012, 4). For a comprehensive study of Jahr's ethics see:

using human subjects. I will not consider issues relating bioethics to ecoethics and zooethics in detail here despite the fact that there are evident connections between human well-being and a healthy environment. Now, let us assume that, in the Ashya case, some scientific experiment could be done and ask how professional bioethicists would deal with it. One could appeal to the predominant theory, that is, the four principles mentioned above. As it is also perhaps wellknown, a key player in establishing this use of "bioethics," that is, as referring to the values related to the development of biomedicine, was *The Kennedy Institute for Ethics*.[9]

Now, it is crucial to recall that, back in the 1970's, a US National Commission was created, which led to the establishment of three *prima facie*, middle level principles for dealing with human subjects of scientific experimentation known as the *Belmont Report*: respect for persons, beneficence and justice. This is what the *Ethical Principles and Guidelines for the Protection of Human Subjects of Research* still prescribes:

- Respect for persons incorporates at least two ethical convictions: first, that individuals should be treated as autonomous agents, and second, that persons with diminished autonomy are entitled to protection. The **principle of respect for persons** thus divides into two separate moral requirements: the requirement to acknowledge autonomy and the requirement to protect those with diminished autonomy. […];
- Persons are treated in an ethical manner not only by respecting their decisions and protecting them from harm, but also by making efforts to secure their well-being. Such treatment falls under the **principle of beneficence**. In this document, beneficence is understood in a stronger sense, as an obligation. Two general rules have been formulated as complementary expressions of beneficent actions in this sense: (1) do not harm and (2) maximize possible benefits and minimize possible harms. […];
- Who ought to receive the benefits of research and bear its burdens? This is a question of justice, in the sense of "fairness in distribution" or "what is deserved." An injustice occurs when some benefit to which a person is entitled is denied without good reason or when some burden is imposed unduly. Another way of conceiving the **principle of justice** is that equals ought to be treated equally.[10]

Muzur, A. & Sass, H.M (eds) *Fritz Jahr and the Foundations of Global Bioethics* (Zürich/Berlin: LIT, 2012).

[9] See Jonsen's book *The Birth of Bioethics* (Oxford: Oxford University Press, 2003, p. 22f) for more details on the history of bioethics, including the role of *The Kennedy Institute for Ethics* to forge the predominant use of "bioethics."

[10] These guidelines are still in place in the US (www.hhs.gov). For a critical discussion on the impact of the *Belmont Report*, see: Childress, J. F. *et al. Belmont*

These principles were mainly applied in the intersection of medical ethics and research ethics, and the *Belmont Report* became a sort of "constitution" of bioethics in the US and around the world. I will refer to this normative framework that contains *respect for persons* (and not just respect for autonomy) as the "Belmont Approach" and argue that it provides, *pace* principlialists, a better basis for neurobio*ethics*.

After the publication of the *Belmont Report*, there was fierce discussion about whether these basic norms were sufficient to deal with all bioethical issues. Many bioethicists doubted that these principles were sufficient to regulate scientific experiments involving human subjects such as Aysha. Perhaps we should add new principles; perhaps we do not need general, formal principles, but casuist analyses of particular cases instead, since there might not be universal norms in bioethics anyway; perhaps we need a criterion to prioritize one of them to solve tensions and even dilemmas; perhaps we need not only principles, but virtues, for instance discernment, to apply these principles well; and so on. I will examine some of these normative alternatives in the next section and in the next chapter.

Despite the fact that bioethics came soon to have an ethical framework to deal with moral problems involved in healthcare practices, *neuro*ethics did not have the same success. It was only after 2002, following the first papers devoted to the neuroethics of moral judgment (Moll, Greene etc.) and a series of meetings in Canada and in the US that an interdisciplinary body of questions emerged.[11] It led Adina Roskies to distinguish two different, but supposedly interconnected, meanings of "neuroethics": on the one hand, the *ethics* of neuroscience (neuro*ethics*) and, on the other hand, the *neuroscience* of ethics (*neuro*ethics).[12] The idea was that neuroscientific studies could not only provide a better understanding of moral phenomena but also better ethical theories to be used in daily life including in doing neuroscience. The main problem, however, is that this seems to presuppose

---

Revisited. Ethical Principles for Research with Human Subjects. Washington: Georgetown University Press, 2005.

[11] To my best knowledge, the first neuroscientific study of moral phenomena using fMRI was done by two Brazilians: Oliveira-Souza, R. & Moll, J. The Moral Brain: functional MRI correlates of moral judgment in normal adults. *Neurology* 2000; 54 (Suppl. 3): 252.

[12] Roskies, A. Neuroethics for the New Millennium. *Neuron,* 2002; 35: pp.21-23. Paramount in establishing the issues of the new field was Martha J. Farah's 2002 paper "Emerging Ethical Issues in Neuroscience," published in *Nature. Neuroscience* 5(11). At that time, Farah argued that "three broad issues survive the triage for novelty and imminence: enhancement of normal function, court-ordered CNS intervention and 'brain-reading.'"

scientificism and even imply moral nihilism. I will discuss this point in the third section bellow and in chapter 3 in greater detail.

The debate on the interfaces between bioethics and neuroethics is as old as neuroethics itself. There are clear classic bioethical issues in neuroethics, but some authors believe that there are also new ethical challenges emerging from neuroscience and neurotechnology. In her introduction to the excellent book *Neuroethics*, Martha J. Farah (2010, 2) asks: *Does the field of neuroethics really need its own name, distinct from philosophy of mind or bioethics?* In her positive answer, which holds that there is more to neuroethics than classic bioethics applied to neuroscience, she assumes that neuroscience gives us unprecedented ways to understand the human mind and *to influence and even to control it*. That certainly is the case, but the ethical question is whether the normative framework based on *respect for persons, beneficence* and *justice* is not sufficient to guarantee the morality of such neuroscientific studies and their neurotechnological applications. It seems clear that the neuroscience of morality itself has not yet produced anything substantially new in normative terms. Therefore, as we will see in chapter 2, recent arguments from Joshua Greene (2017, 11) to establish once and for all utilitarianism as *the* normative ethics evoke skepticism and need to be examined deeply.

After all, what can neuroscience do for ethical theory and, particularly, for meta-ethics? The potential results of the neuroscience of morality cannot be overstated. In a recent paper entitled “Can Neuroscience Contribute to Practical Ethics?” several important neuroethicists redefined the goals of neuroethics from the old ambitious aims into more moderate ones.[13] We are all well aware of Libet’s experiment in the early 1980s, its alleged deterministic implications, and its challenge to the notions of moral responsibility and legal imputation. According to the authors of the paper “Can Neuroscience Contribute to Practical Ethics?” the idea that the neuroscience of ethics could lead to a better or more comprehensive ethical theory, that it could generate a universal morality that transcends cultural divides, that it could be used to develop a brain-based morality etc. are promises that, at this point, neuroscience seems truly unable to deliver. We can see now a turn to more moderate goals and attempts to make less ambitious contributions, such as to inform and enrich ethical analyses and deliberations and verify empirically ethical theories’ main claims. As I pointed out above, fMRI could help us to determine brain injuries (e.g., serious motor, learning or sensory impairments) in order to help us to decide

---

[13] Racine *et al.* Can Neuroscience Contribute to Practical Ethics? *Bioethics* 5(31), 2017, p.331.

what to do in Aysha case. It cannot, however, determine the values involved in the decision-making process without violating Hume's Law (1978, 469-70) or commiting the naturalistic fallacy.[14]

Interestingly enough, such a turn from ambitious goals (whether there is free will or not) to more modest tasks needs to be made using methodological and moral signposts for doing neuroscience of morality. This reveals in fact that it is crucial to advance the *ethics of neuroscience* (Racine *et al.* 2017, 332). These signposts go from the necessity for conceptual and normative transparency (e.g., defining clearly "morality;" outlining the meta-ethical positions underlying the research; etc.) through the search for maximal scientific validity using interdisciplinary methods to reach a balanced interpretation (e.g., hesitating to draw premature conclusions etc.). As can be seen, ethics is guiding good neuroscience not the other way around.[15]

There is no doubt that current topics such as interconnections between moral reasoning and emotions in the formulation of moral judgments, the distinctive neural process that are emblematic to different ethical theories, etc. are worthy of neuroscientific research. My only doubt at this point is whether this research must go under the label of science and not of a subfield of ethics. For instance, Greene's claim (2017, 11) that the neuroscience of morality confirms utilitarianism as *the* ethical theory seems flawed and needs to be carefully examined. First, Greene's criticism of an ethics based on rights seems, as we will see in chapter 2, flawed. Second, many varieties of utilitarianism are not incompatible with rights at all. There are, of course, many versions of consequentialism and much depends on the value theory associated with it. I have no big objections to a sophisticated consequentialist ethical theory such as the one defended by Peter Railton (2003), who, as we will see in the next chapters, spells out a clear list of intrinsic values including deontic notions such as respect for persons. In fact, I will support a hybrid normative approach comprising a reformulation of Parfit's Triple Theory in the direction of a first ethical principle. The discussion on normative ethical theories, however, will come in the next chapter.

---

[14] Hume's Law, which must not be conflated with Moore's naturalistic fallacy, interdicts inferring directly a prescriptive judgment (an *ought* to act) from a descriptive proposition (what *is* the case): any prescription from the workings of "the moral brain" (brain regions such as parts of the prefrontal cortex –VMPFC, DLPFC– and amygdala) implicated in moral judgement about particular values. I will return to this point in chapter 3 in greater detail.

[15] For a general discussion on the ethics of science, see: Resnik, 1998, still one of the best books on this subject.

I can, finally, formulate one of the main points I would like to make in this work, namely that, strictly speaking, there is a misuse of the word "ethics" in the neologism "*neuro*ethics" when we intend to mean a neuroscientific study of morality with normative implications. That is to say, the neuroscience of morality is, as trivial or pompous as it may sound, just neuro-*science*. *Neuro*ethics could, perhaps, be a subchapter of *behavioral* neuroscience, but this is still just a scientific study.[16] Even this, though, can be disputed since most neuroscientific textbooks such as *Neuroscience – Exploring the Brain* do not include any neuroscientific study of moral issues (cf. Bear *et al.* 2016). The only moral issue mentioned in the textbook is whether neuroscientists should use non-human animals in their research. Even when the brain and behavior is examined (Part Three of the manual above), nothing *normative* is stated to deal with patients exhibiting, for instance, mental disorders such as bipolarity, depression, schizophrenia, etc., but only the chemical and biological bases of such disorders. This is, indeed, good *science*, but to do good *ethics* we need something else apart from neuroscience.

Another related point I would like to make is that neuro*ethics*, understood here in its proper sense as *the ethics of neuroscience*, turns out to be just a subfield of bioethics; hence, neurobioethics! If this is right, then neuro*ethics* stands, as neonatal bioethics does, as a specific field of special bioethics. That is to say, neurobioethics is the *ethics* of doing specific scientific studies which use human subjects (for instance, fMRI to understand the role of emotions in moral reasoning) in the neuroscientific field, that is, of what is going on in our nervous system when we judge morally.

To establish neurobioethics, we need to do two things: first, sort out the best bioethical principles; second, check whether there is any moral issue in the ethics of neuroscience (the so-called "neuro*ethics*") not covered by such moral norms. Now, even if this point proves problematic, then it still makes sense to take seriously the idea of *neurobioethics* to deal with the interfaces between traditional bioethics and the new challenges from neuroscience and neurotechnology. As was pointed out above in presenting some of the goals of O3, these may include the new technologies for monitoring and manipulating the brain; the use of psychopharmacology to

---

[16]As it was pointed out by Conrad and von Vries in their work "Field of Dreams: A Social History of Neuroethics" (see references), the neuroscience of ethics is just *science* after all and *neuro*ethics may perhaps have the same destiny as Gen-ethics, that is, a field with no specific subject (2011, p.305). I do agree with Conrad and von Vries that *understanding our ethical faculties is a scientific, not an ethical issue*. Consequently, the neuroscience of ethics should not be part of neuroethics.

change or enhance normal brain functions, etc. General ethical concerns here relate to the value of privacy (especially, privacy of thought), safety in experimental tests, distributive justice and so on. But these seem to be just *classical bioethical issues* after all. Even if they are not or even if one insists on the need for a new name for a new field, there is a case for testing whether neurobioethics can deal with all of them in a proper ethical manner. Why? Because the neuroscience of ethics has apparently failed so far to provide us with a better normative ethics. To decide most neuroethical moral issues, we still need to look for guidance from the best normative framework of bioethics.

1.2 – The main flaws in the predominant bioethical theory

In the previous section, I argued that *neuro*ethics, understood as the neuroscience of morality, has not delivered yet a normative system capable of dealing with practical moral problems including the ones proposed by neuroscientific investigations (e.g., how best to respect persons such as Aysha and her collegues). In fact, the shift from the neuroscience of ethics to the ethics of neuroscience cannot be made, as we will see in the next section, without committing a category mistake. For this reason, neuroethicists need guidance from classical bioethical principles. But, if this is right, the main question is this: which is the proper *normative* framework to deal with the new challenges from neuroscience and neurotechnologies? The neurobioethical point formulated above says we should look for guidance from the traditional bioethical principles, but which ones? For instance, respect *for persons* (Belmont) or just respect for *individual autonomy* (principlism)?

As I mentioned above, after the publication of the 3 *prima facie* principles of the *Belmont Report* there was no consensus regarding the foundations of bioethics. Bioethicists working with particularist methods (e.g., casuistry) held that there are no universal bioethical norms. In their book *The Abuse of Casuistry*, philosopher Albert Jonsen (himself a member of *The National Commission*) and Stephen Toulmin (a Wittgensteinian philosopher) recommended a specific method to analyze cases: (i) pay attention to the morally relevant features of the case; (ii) find paradigmatic cases; (iii) consider the maxim associated with the paradigmatic case and use it to shed light. These are important methodological guidelines, but their application may produce arbitrary solutions and ultimately have relativistic outcomes. Consequently, we may follow such orientations in analyzing cases such as Aysha, but still look for universal principles, for instance, "first, do no harm!" capable of an aprioristic justification to avoid these unethical outcomes.

Casuistry did, however, not become the predominant approach. The most prominent normative theory to deal with bioethical issues came to be the four principles approach or, as dubbed by its critics, "principlism" (or even the "Georgetwon Mantra"). The utilitarian philosopher Tom Beauchamp, out of his own experience at *The National Commission*, and the deontologist James Childress wrote the already mentioned book *Principles of Biomedical Ethics* in 1979. It is a work that has been through several reformulations and editions but that has always kept one basic idea, namely that, in fact, we need 4 rather than the 3 principles quoted above from the *Belmont Report*. Beauchamp and Childress made two important changes in the basic norms of bioethics:

(i) Respect for Autonomy (and not respect for *persons*): one ought to respect *the choices* of subjects of scientific research/patients;
(ii) Non-maleficence (not *beneficence* only): basically, one ought to refrain from inflicting harm.

The principles of beneficence and justice remained roughly the same as stated in the official document reconstructed in the previous section.

According to Beauchamp and Childress, each of these *prima facie* basic norms justifies a set of particular rules *specifying* what must be done in particular circumstances. To illustrate: if your intuition tells you to accept the principle of non-maleficence, then particular rules follow, such as do not kill, do not incapacitate, etc. This can be done for other principles as well, avoiding the traditional objections that the principles are *formal, abstract* and consequently incapable of guiding action. Moreover, one needs to contrast the basic norms and *ponder* which one(s) applies to a specific case, for instance, the Aysha case. Should we respect parents' autonomy by giving them whatever they want or should we avoid, above all, harming the student herself? It is a further question whether pondering is sufficient or whether one needs a kind of metaprinciple capable of unifying all these middle-level principles to evade the moral dilemmas generated by a clash of these fundamental norms. In this regard, Beauchamp and Childress kept the intuitionist meta-ethics of the *Belmont Report* and remained agnostic on the existence of such a Golden Rule. I will deal with this problem soon.

Before critically examining the intuitionist meta-ethical assumptions of the predominant theory, I would like to say that, in Brazil, this bioethical approach became *the official* one despite the strong influence of Catholic bioethics.[17] Until recently, Res. 196/1996 (now updated to 466/2012) stated that ethics in scientific investigations involving human subjects amounts to:

a) freely given and informed consent of target-individuals and the protection of vulnerable groups and the legally disabled (*autonomy*). To that end, research involving human subjects must always preserve their dignity, respect their autonomy and defend them in their vulnerability;
b) weighing risks and benefits, both actual and potential, individual and collective (*beneficence*), making a commitment to maximize benefits and minimize distress and risks;
c) ensuring that predictable injury will be prevented (*non-maleficence*);
d) social relevance of the research, with significant advantages to the research subjects and minimization of the burden to vulnerable individuals, which guarantees equal consideration of all interests involved and preserves the socio-humanitarian purpose of research (*justice and equality*).

As I pointed out above, these principles must be balanced against one another to achieve a proper application. For instance, by considering both non-maleficence and beneficence one should reach a surplus of benefits over harms (symbolizing: B>H), but sometimes, if nothing good results, justifiably refrain from action (¬H). Once again, in the case of the principle of justice, it only states that a fair distribution is an equitable one (that is, equal among equals, differently among unequals; symbolizing: =, =; ≠, ≠), but the material criterion to distinguish what counts as *different or unequal* is open to debate, both in the US's *Belmont Report* and in the four principles approach as well as in the Brazilian document (Res. 466/2012).

There are many problems within the predominant approach. First, some critics have argued that it leads to arbitrary applications. For instance, some Brazilian bioethicists hold that it is open to cultural relativism, which means that, for instance, in the US, the principle of respect for autonomy is generally more applied to solve difficult cases, while, in a developing country, it would make more sense to appeal to *solidarity* or even to justice, leading to a different outcome. Granted, the US is famous for its individualism, but does that imply that one principle has primacy over the

[17] The book *Problemas Atuais de Bioética*, written by Leo Pessini and Christian de Paulo de Barchifontaine (see references), may, keeping in mind the relevant differences, be considered Brazil's equivalent to the *Principles of Biomedical Ethics* in terms of its influence.

other?[18] I do not think so, and classical principlists rightly deny this assumption. There is no doubt that we must be sensitive to transcultural variations in applying principles, but does that imply that North American, Brazilian, Asian, Muslim etc. specific values override basic norms such as *respect for persons*? Does it ethically matter that, in the US, Protestantism is predominant, while in Brazil, Catholicism is? I think that from *descriptive* relativism ("harm" may mean something different here and there) *ethical* relativism does not follow. There are, of course, different kinds of harm, but pain, disability, loss of freedom, etc. are bad in themselves for all members of our lifeform, for all humans. Once again: the basic norms are meant to be universal. We may state them as follows: for all persons, always, it is morally wrong to act in such a way that B<H (less benefits than harms); for all persons, always, it is morally wrong also to distribute rights and obligations in this way =, ≠ (equally among the different or unequally among equals). The cultural variations in applying these principles may, however, be due to their meta-ethical weakness, their intuitionist assumptions, a situation which can, as we will see in the next section, be corrected by practical cognitivism.

It seems clear, then, that the predominant approach does not help to solve the main problems, for instance as represented by the tensions in the care mentioned above. The main reason, in my view, is *the meta-ethical intuitionist basis of principlism itself*. By "intuitionist meta-ethics," I basically mean here the plurality of principles without any ranking order among them or any appeal to a first principle.[19]Astonishingly enough, the authors of *Principles of Biomedical Ethics* recognize that a plurality of middle level norms without a first principle may lead to "irresolvable moral dilemmas" (Beauchamp & Childress 2013, 12). There are countless examples

---

[18] According to Albert Jonsen (2003, 390), the North American *ethos* comprises three facets: moralism, meliorism and individualism, while solidarity is a European value. Since Brazil has a universal socialized health care system (SUS) based on *solidarity*, inspired by the British NHS, many bioethicists hold that we have in Brazil a European bioethics instead of the American one. On this point, for Portuguese (and Spanish) readers see: dos Anjos, M. F. & Siqueira, J. E. (2003); for English readers, see: and Pessini *et al.* (2010). Unfortunately, I cannot in this work make a complete comparison to sort out all the similarities as well as all the differences between American, Brazilian and European bioethics.

[19] I follow here John Rawls' definition (1999, 34), "Intuitionist theories, then, have two features: first, they consist of a plurality of first principles which may conflict to give contrary directives in particular types of cases; and second, they include no explicit method, no priority rules, for weighing these principles against one another." The influence of intuitionism on formatting the principles of bioethics is well known and documented (see Beauchamp & Childress 2013, 15f.)

of conflict between, one the one hand, respect for autonomy and, on the other hand, beneficence or even justice. Aysha case just illustrates these tensions: would be right to satisfy the parents' wishes or should we refrain from doing harm to the student *herself*? Generally speaking, principlism has no clear criterion to decide either way; it not only generates tensions, but "real" moral dilemmas.

This problem seems to be a fatal one for principlism. To clarify, I would like to ask here: what is the logical form of a *real* dilemma? This point is crucial, since I will maintain that there are no real moral dilemmas, only apparent ones. I believe we can represent the logical form of a real dilemma in these terms:

$$(Op \wedge Oq) \wedge \neg \Diamond (p \wedge q)$$

In natural language, it is obligatory to do p (e.g., to respect Aysha's choice) and it is also obligatory to do q (e.g., not to produce more harm than benefits) and it is not possible to do both at the same time.

Now, if dilemmas are not solved, we are left with many tensions, conflicts, etc. in caring practices and, ultimately, *inaction*. The philosophical question, however, is whether *real* moral dilemmas do in fact exist. One may have doubts on this ontological point, but, in any case, an ethical theory cannot generate them because of its unstable meta-ethical foundations, leaving us without any good way out. Beauchamp and Childress' appeal to specification is insufficient to avoid this theoretical difficulty. I believe, however, that an *apparent* dilemma is just due to the *epistemic* limitations of the agent. Of course, there are many tensions in medicine and particularly in neuroscience between seeking to increase *knowledge*, which is a good after all, and protecting the *subject's well-being* (e.g., Aysha), but they are not dilemmas in the ontological sense. I will argue in the next section of this chapter that we do need a new moral epistemology, namely practical cognitivism, to avoid the moral dilemmas generated by the intuitionist meta-ethics of principlism and to show us *how* to respect in a proper way, that is, by expressing a *caring* attitude.

There have been many attempts to avoid the dilemmatic implications of the predominant normative theory in bioethics, but they generate other problems of their own. I would, then, like to mention here one single strategy to overcome the intuitionist meta-ethics of the predominant normative theory *by ranking* one basic norm over the others, with two different outcomes. This basic tactic is simply to prioritize one principle over the others: either autonomy over beneficence or the other way around. Consider, for instance, the physician and philosopher Tristam Engelhardt's principle, which gives always absolute priority to individual consent: "authority for actions involving others in a secular pluralistic society is derived from the free consent of those involved," (1996, 122). Engelhardt's view on the above case would be to give Aysha or to her parents whatever they wanted. The principle of autonomy (or permission) leads to a morality of mutual respect only. Engelhard has, however, a *negative* concept of "respect," which is different from what I will defend here. Now, autonomism appears to solve the dilemmas, but may lead to individualism. In my view, always to give priority to individual autonomy in all circumstances may generate moral indifference and, consequently, a kind of *uncaring* respect. Moreover, as the Kantian philosopher Onora O'Neil correctly pointed out, the emphasis simply on informed consent does not restore public trust in science since it may become ritualistic: people may just sign the informed consent without even read it.[20]

The same strategic method to avoid dilemmas can be employed in a more traditional approach based on the Hippocratic prioritization of beneficence. Here the best account is provided also by a physician and philosopher, namely Edmund Pellegrino.[21] His *beneficence-in-trust model* is based on an Aristotelian assumption, namely a teleological account of the good, which includes autonomy as one of its elements. According to the co-author of the book *For the Patient's Good*, the end to be sought comprises four main ingredients: (i) the patient's clinical good; (ii) her best interest –autonomy–; (iii) her good as a human person; (iv) her view on the ultimate *telos* of life. This approach is the most accepted view among health professionals: it is echoed in The Millennium Physician Charter (2002) and the new Physician's Pledge of the World Medical Association –October 2017– which asserts *the priority* of the patient's well-being over concerns for the patient's individual autonomy.The main problem with this model is, however, that it does not seem to overcome traditional autocratic forms of paternalism which potentially lead to *disrespectful* practices.

I would now like also briefly to discuss the need for prioritization of justice. I know that since I am from a developing country, many would assume that I should put more weight on distributive issues. This was after all the main voice of the congress of the *International Association of*

---

[20] O'Neil, O. *Autonomy and Trust in Bioethics* (Cambridge: Cambridge University Press, 2002). I think that Onora O'Neil is right in criticizing *individual* autonomy, which must be distinguished from the Kantian notion of auto-*nomy*. I will return to this point later.

[21] Pellegrino, E. & Thomasma, D. *For the Patient's Good* (New York/Oxford: Oxford University Press, 1981) 184f.

Bioethics held in Brasília in 2002.[22] Evidently, social issues are crucial, but I will argue that we can in fact *reduce* the principle of justice, meaning basically the right to get one's own share, to be included into the principle of *respect for persons* considering a "person" in the following way: a rights holder and a bearer of obligations. These rights include self-determination, but also *to be cared for* properly in a fair healthcare system, *to obtain an equal share* in a fair distribution etc. This makes it possible to look for the fundamental attitude, namely caring respect, that we are after here. Thus, I will avoid also the introduction of new principles into the basic normative framework, for instance respect for communities or respect for the sanctity of life or any other issue related to justice. I will return to the issue of prioritization while discussing public policies for cognitive enhancers in Chapter 3.

Engelhardt's autonomism and Pellegrino's beneficence-in-trust, then, generate new problems: respect without care may lead to indifference and individualism (uncaring respect); care without respect, to paternalism (disrespectful care). To avoid both at the same time, I believe we need to go back to the core idea of the *Belmont Report*. This means, basically, to stand by the maxim of *respect for persons* instead of just respect for individual autonomy. Moreover, we need to correct its intuitionist assumptions not by prioritizing one principle over the other, but by finding an objective metaprinciple to apply the middle level norms.

A better solution to avoid the tensions in caring for is, then, to find a special kind of norm, a metaprinciple, to guide the application of middle level principles. At this point, I would simply like to mention the two most plausible candidates, namely the Categorical Imperative and the Principle of Utility: Kant's first principle (whose *general* single formula is this: "act only in accordance with that maxim through which you can at the same time will that it become a universal law")[23] and Mill's Greatest Happiness Principle, at least as it appears in the book *Utilitarianism*, which states that "actions are right in proportion as they tend to promote happiness, wrong as they tend to produce the reverse of happiness."[24] Granted, principlists reject

---

[22] The main papers are now published in the following book: Garrafa, V &Pessini, L. (eds). *Bioética: Poder e Injustiça*. São Paulo: Loyola/São Camilo, 2004.

[23] Kant, Immanuel. (GMM4: 421). *Practical Philosophy*. Cambridge: Cambridge University Press, 2008. p.73. The relationship between this general formulation of the Categorical Imperative and the other formulae will be discussed later.

[24] Mill, John Stuart. *Utilitarianism*. Oxford: Oxford University Press, 2011. p.55. Mill's moral theory needs, however, to be reworked in terms of *rule*-consequentialism to be made compatible with a Kantian ethics. This point will be discussed in the next chapter.

this appeal to first principles, perhaps because they are not able to make up their minds on which one is the best candidate. There are, however, many important philosophers working in the direction of overcoming this dichotomy between deontology and consequentialism in normative ethics. These *basic* norms may, then, not be as completely incompatible as it is sometimes believed. Moreover, I think that the most promising attempt to overcome the differences between normative ethical theories was very recently given by the so-called "Triple Theory" presented by Derek Parfit (2013). I will return to the existence or not of a first principle in ethics in the next chapter, which is mainly devoted to *normative* issues.

As I said above, I will now deal with the *meta-ethical* foundations of neurobioethics. Thus, it is crucial to bear the main point in mind: the basic idea is to substitute the intuitionist assumption of the predominant theory to avoid dilemmas and to find a way of *knowing-how* to integrate care and respect. For that, we need a better moral epistemology, namely practical cognitivism. It is worth recalling here that doctors did not *know-how* to apply bioethical guidelines and that is an *epistemic* problem. Let us, then, see whether practical cognitivism can shed some light on what is missing regarding the epistemic basis of bioethics and neuroethics.

1.3– Grounding neurobioethics on practical cognitivism

To start with, I would like to say a few more words on the conception of philosophy I assume here. I take "philosophy," following a Socratic tradition, to be a search for wisdom that has a *protagonist* role in our lives. Now, wisdom is *knowing-how* to apply knowledge, especially scientific, and sound values to act and to live well. In searching for (self)knowledge, wisdom leads to a re-*cognition* of the limits of empirical knowledge, and, at the same time, a rejection of radical skepticism. It also keeps open the possibility of moral knowledge, for instance, of the virtues. It, then, denies different forms of dogmatism such as sophistry and ideologies such as fundamentalisms based on specific worldviews. It follows that only an *agnostic* and finite, that is, a critical ontology is possible, leading necessarily to pluralism, which is not synonymous with normative relativism either. Thus, despite the *agonistic* character of pluralism, we must deal with *a morality* based on sharable grounds while allowing for some differences in beliefs and practices. As we will see presently, such a moral system can be justified from a *cognitivist* point of view.

In this section, then, I will mainly present a meta-ethical theory and outline the main tenets of a new kind of moral epistemology, which I call "practical cognitivism." I will first argue for the thesis that there is moral knowledge and that it is best understood as involving knowing-how. Both practical skepticism and non-cognitivism can and should be rejected. According to a practical cognitivist, moral knowledge cannot be analyzed in the traditional terms of knowing-that only; it also needs knowing-how. The fundamental idea is that one *knows-how* to deliberate morally, *knows-how* to choose the right thing to do, *knows-how* to follow a rule (not only to act in accordance), *knows-how* to react emotionally or even to have appropriate feelings in certain circumstances, *knows-how* to distribute a good, *knows-how* to be a certain kind of person, *knows-how* to give reasons (to justify one's actions), etc. only if one has learned and is *capable of* following the appropriate *normative standards* (in short, norms). I take "norm," in the conceptual analysis of knowing-how, in a very broad sense, to mean a "prescriptive standard," and I will clarify it further soon by discriminating subspecies of norms in order to identify the moral ones.

The first question, then, I should deal with here is this one: what is *moral* knowledge after all? It seems clear that morality is not just a matter of having appropriately *justified true beliefs* (the traditional definition of knowing-that), but, more importantly, in the practical sense, it is being capable of doing something right in practice, perhaps similar to mastering a skill or technique such as handwriting or swimming and so on. These are, of course, non-moral examples of knowing-how. Peter knows-how to ride a bike has no moral import. But *moral* knowing-how is certainly a matter of *acting, being* etc. in certain ways. To illustrate in a more specific way, this is the case when one knows-how to be a certain kind of person, for instance a *caring* and a *respectful* one. These are clearly examples of moral knowing-how. Thus, in order to construct a meta-ethical theory, particularly a new moral epistemology, as a substitute for the intuitionist bases of principlism, I need to specify the differences between *moral* knowing-how and *non-moral* knowing-how. My analysis of knowing-how, which is based on a Wittgensteinian conception of philosophical grammar, reveals, as we will see, that such a kind of knowledge is the result of learning and developing the relevant capabilities.[25] It exhibits also the centrality of norms (principles, rules and other normative standards) for members of our lifeform.[26]

---

[25] For those not familiar with Wittgenstein's philosophy, I would recommend Glock's dictionary (see references) which deals with his main concepts such as language-games, rule-following, family resemblances, hinge propositions, lifeform etc. For more advanced studies, I suggest Peter Hacker's books, especially his commentaries of the PI (cf. references). For those able to read Spanish, see my book *La ética en Wittgenstein y el problema del relativismo* (València: PUV Press, 2016).

[26] I follow here Wittgenstein's point on sharing the human lifeform (*Lebensform*) as a necessary precondition for communication (PI §241). 'Lifeform,' then, is not a

To begin an examination of "knowing-how," it seems necessary to make a distinction between *implicit* (or tacit) and *explicit* knowing-how. *Implicit knowing-how* is an innate capacity, for instance, a baby's ability to nurse. Now, *explicit knowing-how* involves mastering a set of norms, for example riding a bike. Thus, I would now like to analyse under which conditions we may say that a person explicitly knows-how to ride a bicycle.

First of all, she must have been *trained* in some minimal sense to do that, even if it was at the very beginning by observing her father or someone else and trying to mimic their movements. At this stage, training may also include knowing-that such and such. That is to say, propositional knowledge is needed to know-how, although it is not sufficient. Therefore, this distinction between different kinds of knowledge is not meant to introduce a *dichotomy* between the theoretical and the practical (e.g., *Sophia* vs. *phronesis*, EN 1143^{b}15), but if an individual wants to learn to play a new game, let us say, chess, then she must necessarily internalize the norms. It is not enough to read the instructions; she needs to practice too (after all, only *practice* makes perfect). It may be the case that she starts off by being guided until she can play by herself and try to perform the basic moves etc. Some conditioning may well be necessary, but, at some point, she needs to receive instructions on how to proceed autonomously. Consequently, she learns by acting, by doing.

Another condition then is that she learn the required *norms*, both principles and rules, of this activity. Norms may here be taken in a very broad sense: from any action-guiding instruction (even if not verbalized) to explicit normative prescriptions about how to proceed. Thus, in the bike example, she must *learn how* to remain balanced on the vehicle (P_1), *how* to pedal in a synchronized way (r_1), *how* to use the handlebars (r_2), etc. Mastering these norms is essential for knowing-how to practice the activity of riding a bicycle. *Mutatis mutandis*, norms stand in knowing-how for what propositions represent in knowing-that. The apprentice may also at some point be able to re-invent that activity by reforming the rules. It is possible then to be a fallibilist not only about beliefs and justifications of propositions, but also about capacities to follow norms. The same condition applies to practices such as knowing-how to play chess and so on.

---

naturalistic concept, which makes the particularist interpretations of Wittgenstein's ethics held by Toulmin (1986), Nelson (2001) and Little (2001) mistaken. I will, consequently, assume that there are common moral features of the human condition such as empathy, capacity to follow norms etc. See, however, Glock's entry "Form of life" (2005, pp.124-129) for two interpretations, the transcendental and the naturalist readings of *Lebensform*.

Eventually, a person must be *capable of* following and applying the relevant norms(s) by herself and then performing the movements that are constitutive of the very knowledge of how to ride a bicycle. Once she *has learned* how to follow the required norms and has engaged in the activities of the practice a number of times, she may perform in a habitual way the operations that are constitutive of knowing how to ride a bicycle. Thus, one learns and eventually knows-how by doing. Knowing-how becomes part of her "second nature," that is, through education this ability becomes part of her being. She builds up habits through constant training, which is not only mechanical repetition, but may involve (self) criticism as well. This is true of many practices including morality.

It is crucial to be clear on this point: *norms* are not the only ingredient of the moral life, but they are the most objective tool to guide actions. Thus, a practical cognitivist recognizes that a moral system may comprise moral sentiments (sympathy, guilt ...), rights/obligations (right to life; duty not to kill …), emotions (shame …), values (equality, freedom …), character traits (integrity …), etc. Furthermore, a practical cognitivist does not want to reduce all these elements to rules. But norms, for example moral principles such as "Do not cause harm!" or particular rules such as "Do not lie!" do play a central role in guiding our behavior. For one thing, it is by using norms that we usually discriminate *right* (obligatory, forbidden, permissible) actions from *wrong* ones; it is using *principles* that we may justify, that is, give reasons to follow particular *rules*. Recognizing the centrality of norms, then, does not imply that a practical cognitivist supports a deontic rather than an aretaic normative ethics. At this point, though, I will not discuss normative ethics; that is, whether practical cognitivism requires a form of virtue ethics, deontology or consequentialism. I will deal with this issue in the next chapter. The crucial idea to bear in mind right now is that moral knowledge involves *explicit* knowing-how, which was analyzed in terms of having learned and acquiredthe capabilities to follow norms.

Another important point we must keep in mind is that knowing-how is not *reducible* to knowing-that. As I have argued, knowing-that is best defined as having justified true beliefs, while explicit knowing-how is understood as having acquired the capabilities to follow norms. To recognize that knowing-that and knowing-how are *irreducible* to each other is sufficient to put the two definitions of knowledge (A *knows-that* p and A *knows-how* to ϕing) side by side and to realize that the ingredients of one kind of knowing do not appear in the other. A proposition and a norm are different *in kind* and to conflate them is to commit a category mistake; they belong to different language-games. Even if norms can be said to be true, this will be in a different way than propositions are true. This introduces an ontological difference between the existing *facts* and *states of affairs we must bring about* which manifests itself in the linguistic difference between description and prescription, science and ethics, etc. It also does not follow that knowing-how may not have some family resemblances with knowing-that. For instance, sometimes to know *how* to do something is to know the way to do it, and to know the way to do something is often to know that it is done thus-and-so. Therefore, the basic point is just that they represent two different *kinds of knowledge*, which may perhaps be characterized in terms of the traditional distinction between practical and theoretical philosophy. To put it in Humean/Moorean terms: the former deals with what *ought to be*, the latter is an inquiry into what *is* the case; that is, morality cannot be reduced or analyzed in non-moral terms (either natural or metaphysical).

Given that we are mainly discussing the *meta-ethical basis* of neurobioethics here, I would like to bring some evidence from neuroscience to support practical cognitivism. Since the publication of the paper "Cognitive Neuroscience and the Study of Memory" in *Neuron* a few years ago, there has been an intense debate about whether we have non-declarative memory (and not only a declarative record) and its possible association with knowing-how. According to Brenda Milner, Larry R Squire and Eric R. Kandels (cf. references), the development of cognitive neuroscience has, based on studies of a famous case, namely patient H.M., shown that we do not have only declarative (propositional, informational) memory, but, most fundamentally, non-declarative memory, a kind of non-conscious recollection underlying skilled behavior and the ability to respond appropriately to stimuli though practice.[27] Non-declarative memory is the result of conditioning or habit learning and not only of acquiring true or false propositions. According to the authors of the above mentioned study, "… similar ideas had been proposed by philosophers and psychologists on the basis of intuition and introspection. For example, in 1949, Gilbert Ryle, a philosopher of mind at Oxford, proposed the existence of two types of knowledge: *knowing how*, as in knowledge of motor skill and *knowing that*, as in knowledge of fact and event." (1998, 449) Leaving aside whether Ryle

[27] Declarative memory relates to facts and events; nondeclarative memory, to skills, habits, emotional responses, etc. For an updated presentation of memory systems, including an examination of types of declarative and non-declarative memory relating them to the patient H.M. see: Bear *et al. Neuroscience – Exploring the Brain* (Philadelphia: Woters Kluwer, 2016), 824f. I believe patient H.M. shows that knowing-how is *irreducible* to knowing-that. This is a good example of how neuroscience, which is a descriptive and explanatory enterprise, can help in *meta-ethical* discussions which are also descriptive, but not in *normative ethics*.

was relying on intuition only or applying a Wittgensteinian method, that is, doing a grammatical, conceptual investigation on fundamental epistemic verbs such as "to know" (cf. IF, §150-1), it is clear that he was, in the second chapter of his book *The Concept of Mind* entitled "Knowing How and Knowing That," pointing to two *kinds* of knowledge and not only a subtype of the same cognitive phenomenon (knowing *how, when, where* etc.). Thus, it seems that the criticism Bennet and Hacker addressed in their book *Philosophical Foundations of Neuroscience*, namely that knowledge is akin to *being able to*, but it is not another kind of knowledge, that is, *knowing how*, overlooked the fundamental differences between declarative and non-declarative memories. They accused Ryle of committing an error (Bennet & Hacker 2003,155), namely of assuming that knowing-how is never the same as knowing that. But it is unclear whether this thesis, recently developed also by Jason Stanley, in his book *Know How*, is not flawed. If my previous analysis of "knowing-how" is sound, then it supports Ryle's Wittgensteinian distinction.[28] That is to say, knowing-how presupposes memory without conscious record like, for instance, when we act prudently; it is the result of habit, as any moral virtue is and not of having justified true beliefs only. The clear evidence for this claim is patient H.M. himself: "… he learned to perform new tasks despite the fact that he had no recollection of the specific experiences in which he was taught to do them (the declarative component of the learning." (Bear *et al.* 2016, p.842). Therefore, *pace* Bennet and Hacker, we must keep the distinction between two language-games here despite some resemblances: one is propositional and the other nonpropositional. Even if there are some family resemblances between knowing-how and knowing-that, they are irreducible to each other. By the way, the Portuguese language has two words for these two different cognitive phenomena, namely "conhecimento" (from Latin, *cognoscere*) and "saber" (from Latin, *sapere*), which unfortunately we cannot make full sense of using only the English distinction between knowing-how and knowing-that. To know in the *sapere* sense (which can be translated as "having a taste") presupposes *experience*, not only true beliefs. Moral knowledge is a form of "saber," not "conhecimento," that is, of knowing-how. This difference is crucial for a practical cognitivist.

[28] At this point, it might be objected that one may know-how, for instance to ride a bike, but is currently *unable* to do it. This was also raised by Professor Fred Gifford during the conferences at the MSU. Thus, I would like to refine my previous analysis of knowing-how and point out that the third condition cannot be "P is capable of ϕing," but rather "P has learned to ϕing." This revision will also become apparent in my analysis of 'knowing-how to respect' in the third section of the next chapter.

It is for this reason that I have called for a fundamental change in the way we do meta-ethics nowadays, especially moral epistemology. Most present-day debates start with the single and, in my view, wrong assumption that either there is moral knowledge or there is not, but both sides take knowledge only in terms of knowing-that. Consider, on the one hand, the cognitivist meta-ethical theory "classical intuitionism," that is, the thesis that moral knowledge is not empirical, not based on observations, etc. and that it depends on a special faculty, namely intuition, to grasp non-natural moral properties, for instance, the intrinsic goodness of a certain state of affairs. There is a grain of truth in this, but, if radicalized, it leads to categorical errors. For example, G. E. Moore, David Ross and neo-intuitionists alike (especially, today, Robert Audi and David McNaughton) find themselves postulating queer entities and strange faculties to grasp *self-evident* moral facts. Now, on the other hand, Wittgenstein, in his first book, declared, "there are no propositions in ethics" (TLP 6.42), but he had a reductivistic conception of a "proposition," that is, it should be a representation of a state of affairs and, if true, *should picture* a fact in an isomorphic way. Now, this led to the non-cognitivist (if not irrationalist) thesis held by logical positivism: moral judgements are equivalent to pure emotional expressions only such as "Boo!" The shared mistake between intuitionists and emotivists, including other recent forms of expressivism (e.g., Gibbard and Blackburn's quasi-realism), is to assume one kind of knowledge only, either to affirm (most cognitivists) or to deny (non-cognitivists) moral knowledge. That is why I have called for turning the meta-ethical debate in the direction of knowing-how.

It is time now to add some more tenets to this moral epistemology. At this point, then, it seems clear that there are different subspecies of knowing-how, that is, *moral* (caring, respecting etc.) and *non-moral* (riding a bike, playing the piano etc.) ones. Thus, I will now stipulate a particular sense of the word "moral," which is the focal meaning when referring to *a common* and *sharable* morality (*a* CS-Morality). I will develop the main tenets of this morality in the next chapter. Normally, the word "moral" is, in the sciences (including the neurosciences) used as a synonym for "altruist behavior" and stands in opposition to pure self-interest or egoism. This is anyway the predominant use in some scientific domains engaged with morality such as ethnology, sociobiology, psychology, etc. This, however, leaves out the possibility of moral attitudes towards the agent herself. For example, it excludes self-care and self-respect as fundamental obligations. Thus, I would, for *a* CS-Morality, like to use the word "moral," associated with knowing-how, in this sense: it involves an *intrinsic valuation,* and, when two values are at stake, *the overridingness of the moral ones*.[29] Acting rightly (not doing what is forbidden, fulfilling one's own obligations, etc.) presupposes an intrinsic valuation: knowing-how to take care requires doing good to a vulnerable individual because this is best *for her*. Altruistic actions are one instantiation of this kind of valuation, but they are not the only one. For instance, when one cares about oneself, one may also be showing moral concern. On the other hand, when a person does good for other people out of *pure* self-interest, but not because this is good *for* the other person, she does not act morally. In the context of practical cognitivism, from now on, I will take this particular sense of "moral" as presupposing an intrinsic valuation in order to construct *a* CS-Morality as a condition to make present day pluralism reasonable. This is not, obviously, the only possible meaning of "moral," but it is the one that I will use here.

I would briefly like to recall that this intrinsic valuation has been the domain of morality since Aristotle's conception of *praxis*, Kant's definition of "a categorical imperative" as a practical law commanding an action as good in itself, and Wittgenstein's notion of "absolute value." The difference between *making* and *doing* in Aristotle's *Nicomachean Ethics* is plain enough: "For while making has an end other than itself, action cannot; for good action itself is its end." (EN 1140^{b}) The actions of making a house have extrinsic value: the product is the end that justifies them. Now, this is not the case with good actions. Moral actions, character traits, etc. have to do with what is good or bad in itself; for example, murder is bad in itself. Here we see that particularist readings of Aristotle's ethics seem mistaken. Anyway, moral virtues are worth having for their own sake and may be expressions of knowing-how to act morally.

Now, *mutatis mutandis*, one can find the very same idea in Kant's moral philosophy. When Kant discriminates categorical from hypothetical imperatives, he defines the former in these terms: "the categorical imperative would be that which represented an action as objectively necessary of itself, without reference to another end." (GMM 4: 414) Some examples here could be keeping promises, helping people in need, etc. Thus, leaving aside the differences between Aristotle and Kant (e.g., whether we need *good will* to guide the virtues), they would agree on this point: morality is the domain of actions that are good/right in themselves. It is worth stating here what I call "the non-priority thesis;" that is, that both "good" and "right" can be defined in terms of value, and, in the moral case, in terms of *intrinsic* value.

---

[29] For a discussion on the overridingness thesis see: cf. Hare, 1981; 2002.

Before concluding that this view is absolutely incompatible with consequentialism in normative ethics, we need to discuss differences between, for instance, act- and rule- forms of such a normative ethics. It may also be the case that a sophisticated form of consequentialism can make room for saying that an act can be *prima facie* good in itself but must also be judged for its results. This would be the case if, for example, we take the whole of actions and consequences as an organic one. One instantiation of the principle of organic unities is that the value of a pair of shoes is not just the sum of the value of each shoe. If you lose one, no one will buy the other for half the price of the pair. Thus, a Moorean principle of organic unities, that is, the idea that "the value of a whole must not be assumed to be the same as the sum of the values of its parts" (PE, 79), gives us a way of taking the value of the pre-act elements (e.g., intentions) *and* the value of the action itself (whether it is *prima facie* good or right in itself) *and* the values of the results (whether it produces more good despite being *prima facie* wrong) into consideration to establish whether it is the action to be performed. I will develop this idea in the next chapter, when I propose a way of overcoming the normative polarization between virtue ethics, consequentialism and deontology.

In his *Lecture of Ethics*, Wittgenstein makes the distinction between a *relative* and an *absolute* use of moral words such as "good," "right," etc. It reminds us of the Aristotelian distinction between *poiesis/praxis* and the Kantian differentiation between hypothetical/categorical imperatives. Wittgenstein's example is this: suppose I tell you, "You played tennis badly," you can certainly reply, "Ah, that's all right, I was just doing some exercise." But now suppose I had told one of you a preposterous lie and you came up to me and said, "You're behaving like a beast" and then I were to say, "I know I behave badly, but I don't want to behave any better", could you then say, "Ah, then that's all right"? Certainly not; you would say, "Well, you ought to want to behave better". Given that Wittgenstein never refused this criterion in his later philosophical work (it is also in the TLP (6.422)), I will employ it to distinguish moral rules from non-moral ones.[30] Therefore, it seems clear that a moral norm expresses an *intrinsic valuation*, for instance, whether an action, a character trait, etc. is good in itself.

In order to make the distinction between moral and non-moral knowing-how clearer, it may be worth presenting some illustrations. Thus, I would like now to *exemplify* how such moral knowledge instantiates

---

[30] More recently, Ernst Tugendhat (1994), who had a strong influence on my way of doing philosophy, following a Wittgensteinian method of clarifying the meaning of moral terms, also maintained that there is a *grammatically absolute* use of moral terms, despite the fact that he had a less clear criterion to identify them.

important moral attitudes, which will be used as the main cornerstones for *a* CS-Morality, namely caring and respecting. A practical cognitivism should be capable of showing that caring in a respectful way presupposes *moral* knowing-how. To achieve this goal, I would like to recall the case presented in the first section of this chapter to illustrate this point. We should know not only basic scientific facts, but, most importantly, we must *know-how* to take care and to respect Aysha *for her own sake*. This has been clearly pointed out by many care ethicists, so I will elaborate a detailed discussion involving the so-called "care ethics" in the next chapter. The same may be true of other fundamental moral notions such as *respect*: it may involve not only a feeling, for instance of empathy, but effectively knowing-how to *re-cognize* an individual as a person (e.g., as an agent who is a bearer of rights and responsibilities).

It seems plain that we should then consider caring and respecting *attitudes* (comprising internalized norms and proper motivation), as expressions of knowing-how and not only knowledge of facts or information. This means also that I am, from a meta-ethical point of view, assuming internalism as the best moral psychology for explaining morality. That is to say, taking into consideration how moral knowledge is acquired, a practical cognitivist would say that if a person knows-how to educate morally, then she will motivate others to do what is right for its own sake. Consider how we may learn how to respect: a caring attitude may be part of our motivation to do so. Moral education then becomes central and virtue ethicists (and care theorists) have rightly pointed out the importance and power of the example in moral training. It now becomes clear why we need a cognitivist approach in moral epistemology to ground caring respect answering the following question: does one *know-how* to respect (or not), that is, in a caring manner? As we will see, practical cognitivism provides objective support for *a* CS-Morality and may have important implications in applied ethics, that is, in neonatal bioethics, in neurobioethics, etc. I will expand on this in chapter 3.

In what sense does one know-how to care for a vulnerable individual or know-how to respect a person? The knowledge implicit in caring for a vulnerable individual (a human being or a sentient nonhuman animal) is knowing-how, for instance, to increase her well-being *for her own sake*. This is not only in the technical sense of doing what must be done to cure her if she is sick, but it is also in the *moral* sense, which presupposes an intrinsic valuation: the person's well-being must be fostered because it is good *for the patient's* own sake. If there is no such evaluative attitude, there is no moral worth in caring for her. Here, we must also remember that there is a distinction between *natural* care (perhaps out of sympathetic concern only) and *moral* care (established as an obligation). Thus, knowing-how to act morally involves an intrinsic valuation: a person knows-how to care if she answers in the appropriate way, for example sympathetically, to an individual's well-being and acts accordingly to protect it, foster it and so on, doing whatever is necessary.The same reasoning applies to respect. I will develop these points in the next chapter in greater detail.

We have now the main tenets of practical cognitivism. Thus, having made a distinction between moral and non-moral knowing-how, I would like to deal with some more epistemic issues surrounding it. One of these issues is the problem of establishing how objectivity is explained by this new moral epistemology. Now, since norms are said to be the central ingredient of knowing-how to act morally, it seems clear that the discussion of whether moral judgments are objective or not should be related to the kind of entity they are. In this sense, it is not difficult to recognize that norms are objective in their own way; that is, if they are clearly formulated, then they co-ordinate the behavior of all agents. Consider first a non-moral example: traffic rules guide the actions of all drivers around the world; now consider a moral example: keep your promises. This rule may be equally justified, and then followed by all persons, so how can we establish its objectivity? It seems clear that to say "all persons must keep their promises" does not express subjective feelings, but prescribes objectively a specific kind of behavior. It settles an objective standard to say whether an agent acts accordingly. Thus, objectivity in ethics has nothing to do with postulating queer entities existing "out there," which supposedly must correspond to moral terms or concepts. On the contrary, it is a matter of recognizing whether moral norms sufficiently guide behavior. Consequently, moral norms are objective in this sense and once they are internalized, they convert into *attitudes*, which are not subject simply to one's own valuations, for instance, taking care of a teenager *respectfully*.

A crucial distinction needs to be made at this point. As Wittgenstein pointed out in his later work, there is a difference between *following a rule* and *merely acting in accordance with it* (PI §143f.).[31] Mere behavioral conformity with a rule is no guarantee that the agent understands it and that she is really acting accordingly. That is to say, grasping what should be done and actually doing it is a necessary condition to attribute real action and not mere reactions to an agent. If this distinction is not taken seriously, it is not possible to make an agent accountable for her deeds.

---

[31] I have discussed elsewhere (2016, pp.105-7) other fundamental tenets of practical cognitivism inspired by Wittgenstein's remarks on rule-following (PI, §184-243) such as the idea of *hinge moral* propositions, the specificity of *moral* language-games: imperative, evaluative, performative etc.

Thus, according to a practical cognitivist, only following a rule is a real cognitive state. A norm is objective if it makes us *go on doing the same thing* and there are impartial ways of checking whether this is the case.

A practical cognitivist must also investigate whether moral judgements can be said to be true or false. Now, norms may, in some sense, be said to be true or false, but we must make explicit in which sense. According to a Wittgensteinian grammatical investigation on "truth," it seems clear that this concept has many different meanings: either a *correspondence* between a proposition and a fact or the *coherence* within a normative system between principles and rules etc. Thus, it is important to bear in mind here what is, for some uses of "true," established in the §136 of *Philosophical Investigations*, namely:

'p' is true = p; 'p' is false = not-p.

That is to say, "truth" can have different meanings, but it is mistaken to assume that one (e.g., correspondence) can give the whole grammar of how we use the word. It means either correspondence or coherence depending on the moral language-game in which we are contextualizing our moral judgement.

This is perhaps the best place to introduce some differences between moral and non-moral language games. Wittgenstein gave us some illustrations in the famous §23 of the *Philosophical Investigations*: crisscrossing scientific language-games such as forming and testing a hypothesis or presenting the results of an experiment in tables and diagrams with non-scientific ones such as thanking, cursing, greeting, praying, etc., leads to category mistakes, which must be explained away by philosophical analysis. Now, Bennet and Hacker (2010, 68f.) have already pointed out many mereological fallacies that cognitive neuroscientists commit by trying to reduce epistemic explanations to what is going on in our brian. Moreover, I have also developed (2016, 104f.) Wittgenstein's notion to show that there are imperative moral language-games, evaluative moral language-games, performative moral language-games, etc. in order to argue that each region of moral language has its own standards of meaning and truth and cannot be conflated with the rules of other non-moral language games. What cannot happen, then, is to transpose from a *scientific* activity, such as describing neuroscientifically what is going on in our "moral brain," to what is needed for an ethics of doing neuroscience. Much more is necessary to establish a principle like respect for persons than neuroimages. I will return to this pont while discussing Farah's view that personhood is an illusion of the brain.

As we have seen, practical cognitivism relies on the idea that knowing-how involves mastering the application of norms or prescriptive standards. Thus, I would like now to clarify further the *role* norms play in our practices, in our moral life. First of all, it is necessary to keep in mind the difference between *principles* and *rules* without pretending to construct a full typology of norms here. Principles are general or universal standards to guide behavior, while rules are the specification of particular actions. A clear example can be given in neurobioethics where the principle of non-maleficence (*first, do no harm*) justifies particular rules such as "do not kill", "do not cause pain or suffering", "do not cause offense" etc. Thus, norms are objective in the sense that they regulate intersubjective behavior. As we have seen, norms do play a fundamental role in *guiding* a person's behavior, in discriminating *right* from *wrong*, in *justifying* or in giving reasons for actions and so on. Now, since culture, and morality as part of it, is norm-constituted all the way down, it also seems clear that there are all sorts of rules: rules of games, legal rules, etc. There are indeed moral rules, and moral life itself may be better seen as a rule-governed practice in its most objective ingredients. This does not mean that I am committing myself to the view that the moral life exclusively comprises rules. Once again: a moral system may indeed also include sentiments, character traits, values etc. Not all these elements need to be explained by reference to rules or be reduced to them. Norms are, however, necessary for holding persons accountable.

Norms may be objective and even true (in a coherentist sense), but that is not to say that a moral system is not revisable. A practical cognitivist is a fallibilist, not a strong foundationist, in the question of moral justification. As for beliefs, we may constantly revise our set of norms, correcting them, perfecting them as we go along. Knowing-how comes at various levels. Suppose Peter knows-how to drive a car, he can of course improve the way he does this by learning new norms. There are normative standards: drive well; do not drive badly, etc. Consider also whether this is not the case in ethics. For example, the principle of non-maleficence may well be rewritten in terms of "do no more harm than benefit" asking *the research subject herself* (e.g., Aysha) to establish what counts in terms of harm, thus introducing autonomous choices. The rules related to it may also be rewritten and improved. This adjustment is an ongoing project. Consequently, a practical cognitivist is in a better philosophical position as a fallibilist, which may be compatible with a *soft* form of foundationism (there may be basic moral norms after all), but not a strong one (these basic norms are not absolutely irreversible).

This raises the question of whether a practical cognitivist is a realist in meta-ethical terms. Given the results of this section, a strong form of realism needs to be rejected as philosophically unsound. At first sight, then, a practical cognitivist may be considered realist in the *relational* sense only. That is to say, a practical cognitivist may well subscribe to what Peter Railton calls "an objectified subjective interest" for an individual A^+. This is compatible with the conception of philosophy sorted out previously. To quote Railton (2003, 11) in order to clarify better the distinction between A and A^+: "give to an actual individual *A* unqualified cognitive and imaginative powers, and full factual and nomological information about his physical and psychological constitution, capacities, circumstances, history, and so on." Then, what counts as real (e.g., the ingredients of one's welfare) is what is established from the point of view of A^+ and not from a mind independent realm of values. Our moral ontology can then be deflated: there are no strange, queer moral properties "out there". Now, I would like to add another component to Railton's view: A^+ must have *knowing-how* to a high, excellent degree. That is to say, knowing-how presupposes having learned and exercised the capacities in order to act morally or have the appropriate attitudes. Therefore, a practical cognitivist is a realist in the relational sense only as Aristotle, Kant and Wittgenstein arguably were.

To summarize: in this first chapter, I analyzed the interfaces between bioethics and neuroethics and presented a new moral epistemology to overcome the meta-ethical problems of the intuitionist basis of the predominant normative approach, namely principlism. To illustrate this point, I reconstructed the basic facts of the Aysha case. It showed that we still do not *know-how* to care and to respect her properly. That is why I presented a new moral epistemology to try to overcome this state of affairs. Caregivers should *know-how* to take care of vulnerable individuals better and to respect persons properly. To fully overcome the intuitionist basis of the Belmont approach, however, I need to state *a first ethical principle* to guide the applications of the middle level neurobioethical norms. I will do this in the next chapter on normative ethics.

CHAPTER 2

NORMATIVE ETHICS: INTEGRATING CARE AND RESPECT

The general aim of this chapter is to present some of the main tenets of *a* moral system capable of integrating care and respect, two expressions of knowing-how to *intrinsically value* a vulnerable individual or a person (e.g., Aysha), into a coherent whole. I named this value system "*a* common and sharable morality (CS-Morality)," and it is connected to the practical cognitivism developed in the previous chapter with important applications in neurobioethics. This chapter will then be a response to question 6 raised in the introduction: Is there a universal morality that should guide normative judgments about interventions to improve moral behavior and decision-making? By proposing *a* CS-Morality based on mutal care and reciprocal respect, I will briefly answer also the other neurobioethical questions, namely how decisions affecting the mind should be made, the role of criminal justice (neurolaw), how care is constituted when it is delivered via an algorithm or a robot, etc. *A* CS-Morality cannot, however, be conflated with Gert, Culver and Clouser's conception of *the* common morality eventually incorporated into principlism by Beauchamp and Childress. The best evidence that there is no such morality, at least not in the way they conceived it, is their view on stopping food and fluids as the best method for allowing a patient to die (Gert, Culver and Clouser 1997, 292). That is why I prefer to speak in terms of *a* CS-Morality; not, *the* morality.

The predominant normative approach in bioethics is, as we saw in the previous chapter, composed of four principles, which can, as we will see now, be *reduced* to the concepts of care and respect. The principles of respect for autonomy (or the right to self-determination) and of justice (the right a fair share in a distribution) can easily be reduced to the notion of respect for persons as stated in the Belmont Report. The principles of non-maleficence and beneficence can be reduced to the notion of care. The theoretical task afterwards is, then, to integrate care and respect into a coherent moral system: *a* CS-Morality. By simplifying our normative framework, we can apply it more easily *knowing-how* to take care of someone in a respectful way or respect a person in a caring manner. In this chapter I will then construct the concept of *caring respect* and apply it to some issues in neurobiethics, for instance, to students with cognitive problems.

Now, it seems clear that *neuro*ethics, in the sense of the neuroscience of morality, has until now failed to deliver a universal morality. One reason, as I pointed out in the last chapter, may be due to its scientificist assumptions. To illustrate, think of some recent developments in *neuro*ethics driven by naturalism. Does it matter what is going on in one's brain to prove the truth of, for example, hedonism as an ethical theory, that is, the view that *only* pleasure is intrinsically valuable and right actions are the ones leading to it? Of course, brain-imaging shows that the dopamine system is involved in every kind of enjoyment, but should we stimulate it to release endorphins and encephalins or should we do the right thing (e.g., take just our fair share) even if it does not maximize pleasure? Should we not condemn a rapist or pedophile even though they take great pleasure from their acts? The answer is, of course, positive, and it shows that ethics is not an empirical, scientific enterprise only. Thus, it begs the question of whether hedonism is true to measure the level of serotonin or dopamine in one's brain when involved in pleasant activities. Apart from pleasure, perhaps virtue and knowledge are also intrinsically valuable. Perhaps only persons are intrinsically valuable. These are *ethical*, that is, *normative* questions (relative to what we *ought to do*), not factual ones relating to what is the case (how the state of affairs *are*). Therefore, the difference in kind between *normativity* and *factuality* is another way of distinguishing ethics from the sciences (including neuroscience). I will return to these points while discussing the failures of current neuroscientists (e.g., Greene, Farah etc.) in establishing utilitarianism as the true normative ethics.

To achieve the main goal of this chapter, the *problem* I would like to address here is this: under which necessary and hopefully sufficient conditions can we say that W *knows-how* to respect Y in a *caring* manner? That is to say, I will use the meta-ethical theory sorted out in the last section to help us to see clearly how to apply in neurobioethics the normative network provided by the *Belmont Report* while avoiding both the problems of intuitionist assumptions and the difficulties of prioritizing either autonomy or beneficence. I have already pointed out the main problems with the current analysis of "care"; for instance, Nodding's analysis which is circular, states non-necessary conditions, etc. It is, consequently, necessary to re-examine "care" and state when it is respectful.

2.1 –Taking care of the vulnerable

Before looking for the interconnections between caring and respecting, I will, in this first section, re-examine what "care" means and connect it to respect through practical cognitivism, that is, through the meta-ethical thesis that one must *knows-how* to care. Aysha case will guide us since it seems clear that she is a teenager still needing not only respectful care, but beginning to demand caring respect too.

To begin with, I would like to say that one of the most philosophically significant approaches to care I came across is Darwall's Rational Theory of Welfare (RTW). The basic idea of such a theory is that caring for someone is wanting her welfare for her own sake and that a person's good is constituted not necessarily by what that person values, prefers, or wants (or should value), but by what one (perhaps she herself) should want *insofar as one cares about her* (Darwall 2004, 4). This is the core thesis of the RTW which holds that care gives us agent-neutral reasons to act.[32] In this regard, the RTW seems compatible with some forms of consequentialism. Moreover, it is supported by an Aristotelian thesis, namely that a life of virtuous activity is best *for the person herself*, is what benefits *her* most (2004, 82). I have, however, argued that this characterization of care as giving us agent-neutral reasons to act needs further scrutiny, since, as it stands, it may lead to misunderstandings and to paternalistic actions and practices. Granted, virtues are intrinsically valuable, but is there *the* good life composed of the same virtues for everyone? What would be a good life for Aysha? It is not always clear how Darwall manages to integrate care and respect into a coherent moral view that avoids paternalism. In this section, then, I will re-examine the meta-ethical and normative characterizations of the RTW, clarifying in which sense care gives us agent-neutral reasons for action.

There is no doubt that we humans are, as social beings, care-dependent creatures. This is true of other non-human animals too, but our degree of dependence on care seems higher than any other living being. That is to say, from the very moment we are born, or even before that, we need all sorts of care to fulfil our *basic necessities* in order to survive: we must be fed, clothed, protected from many kinds of harm, and so on. Thus, care seems to be above all a response to the basic necessities of a vulnerable being. Now, as infants, we need to *learn how* to become a complete,

[32] According to Darwall (2004, 127), reasons for acting that are rooted in respect are *agent-relative*, while reasons for caring are *agent-neutral*. Darwall is right in the positional sense of "agent-relativity," but as we will see soon, there is a sense in which reasons for acting rooted in respect are agent-neutral too.

autonomous human being by walking, talking, playing, socializing, etc. all activities mastered –or not– through practice and other forms of educational care. Again, this is perhaps true of other animals, especially monkeys. As teens, recalling Aysha, we need to *learn how* to become independent, for instance, to choose our lifestyle, plan a project, make a living, etc. Even as adults, as autonomous agents, we should not only care for those in need, but we should constantly look after ourselves, so self-care is still vital to us. Later in life, most of us will probably become very vulnerable and will need to be cared for again. That is why, as the ancient fable by Hyginus reveals to us, we owe our entire *being* to *Cura*.[33]Consequently, care should be considered a fundamental ethical tenet of *a* CS-Morality based on what is common to all members of our lifeform.

We humans simply owe our *being* to care. This idea was recently pointed out by Virginia Held (2006, 3) and other care theorists against those claiming the absolute priority of the right or the primacy of respect or justice. As we will see presently, however, we do not need to consider care ethics a particular gender-based approach to moral phenomena or just a specific set of duties owned by some professionals only. Care is, as Wittgenstein would put it, grounded in the conditions of our lifeform. Perhaps justice has another kind of primacy, for instance, political, but care is *simply* constitutive of our lifeform. Thus, *care relates to vulnerable individuals; respect, to persons*. There is no contradiction in asserting both and insisting on the idea that care and respect *limit* and, at the same time, *complement* each other in attitudes such as *respectful care* for vulnerable individuals and *caring respect* among persons.

To avoid empty generalizations, however, we must distinguish different kinds of care and look for the moral dimension of caring for a vulnerable individual. To say that "caring may be defined most generally as feeling or showing concern for something or someone" (Engster 2009, 21) does not help much. If we define care in generic terms only, as *Cura*, then it looks like an all-encompassing attitude towards everything, that is, objects, vulnerable individuals, etc., but one that says little about what to do in particular circumstances, for example, in specific neurobioethical contexts. A caring person would care for everything, but in what sense? Thus, what exactly do we mean by the term "care"? To answer this question, I need to make some more distinctions.

One important distinction to avoid confusion is to differentiate between *caring for*, in the sense of *to take care of* someone, and *caring*

[33] In this work, I will use the concept of "human lifeform" as depending on care. (For a discussion on the Wittgensteinian concept of lifeform (*Lebenform*) see: Glock, 2005 and Hacker 2013).

about. It is in this context that one can say that she does not care about whether it rains on her way home. I will return this point soon. As we can see, however, *knowing-how* to take care of someone involves having apt feelings (e.g., sympathy), and being focused on *her* well-being in a certain way, that is, doing it *for her own sake*. It depends on an intrinsic valuation in order to have moral worth. Taking care of someone, consequently, is a *moral* practice; that is, it involves not only capabilities, but becomes a social and political institution. Parenting, teaching, curing and so on are *caring* practices. Consequently, in this work, I am most interested in what it means *to take care of* and not only the nature of caring about.

It is, then, in this context that we can also distinguish between *natural* and *moral care*. Noddings made a clear distinction between *natural* care and *ethical* or *moral* care in these terms: a mother's caretaking on behalf of her child may not usually be considered ethical, but only natural since it is based on sympathy. Ethical caring, according to her, has its origin in a second sentiment, in a memory of our own best moments of caring and being cared for, as an "I must." In her own words: "Kant has identified the ethical with that which is done out of duty and not out of love, and that distinction in itself seems right." (2003, 80). According to her, an ethics built on caring strives to maintain this caring attitude, and it is thus dependent upon, and not superior to, natural caring. For this reason, she may well avoid the naturalistic fallacy of inferring moral obligations from natural phenomena. Thus, I plainly agree also with Virginia Held when she writes that the concept of care should not "… be a naturalized concept and the ethics of care should not be a naturalized ethics." (2006, 39)[34] How to justify the obligation to care is a further issue, but we can here appeal to a *first principle* of ethics, which I will present in the last section of this chapter. As can be seen, moral care (not natural) is based on an *obligation*, and, consequently, it is paramount to uncover the norm(s) underlying such an attitude, which, as we have seen, expresses also a form of knowing-how as analyzed earlier. Among all these kinds of care, we might perhaps say that there are only family resemblances in the use of the word "care".

Perhaps this is the best place to scrutinize some recent neuroscientific attempts to extract a normative ethics. As we will see, this

---

[34] Here we can, one more time, see why neuroethics, in the sense of the *neuroscience of morality*, cannot deliver us a *normative* ethics, namely because of its naturalistic assumptions. Despite Greene's definition of "morality" (2013, 329), moral philosophy *is not* a manifestation of moral psychology. It is for this and other reasons that Bennett and Hacker would be right in saying that Greene's proposition (2013, 59), namely "morality is the human brain's answer to this challenge [cooperation]" is another good example of a mereological fallacy.

naturalistic view misrepresents the nature of morality. Consider this definition as an illustration:

> Morality is a set of psychological adaptations that allow otherwise selfish individuals to reap the benefits of cooperation. (Greene 2013, 23)

According to the author of the book *Moral Tribes*, humans' biological make up favors in-group cooperation (I-We relations), but our moral brains did not evolve in such a way for groups to cooperate with one another (We-Them). That is why universal cooperation seems inconsistent with the principles governing evolution by natural selection.

This is, however, too narrow a definition and an unconvincing explanation of morality. Actually, Greene's definition of "morality" has many other problems: first, it is reductionist since it is based on *psychological* concepts only; second, cooperation is not the only function of morality; third, it cannot make sense of duties to oneself, for instance self-care and self-respect. In the Introduction, I assumed a better definition of morality taken from Crisp's work. Moreover, Greene accepts a utilitarian value system (hedonist) only, which cannot work as a metamorality to overcome the gap between We and Them. *Pace* Greene, Human Rights is the *lingua franca* of contemporary morality. For this reason, I suggested the O3 Group to adopt provisionally a Human Rights approach to work as a metamorality. Evolution is one possible explanation of the origins of a morality, but there are others: religion, philosophical reflection, etc. could also be reasonable sources of moral values. Actually, most *modern* ethical theories are the products of philosophical reflection on natural or human rights. We must, then, take seriously present-day pluralism and work out *a* CS-Morality.

Greene's criticism of a morality based on universal rights is simply ungrounded, as is his appeal to utilitarianism.[35] Besides, Greene neglects the fact that moral and legal rights are not incompatible with a

---

[35] What Greene calls "Trolleyology" (2013, 105) is an interesting way of testing our moral intuitions, but we cannot assume straight away that the utilitarian answer is the correct one. In this sense, what Greene does is interesting *to explain*, using psychology and the neuroscience of ethics, what is going on in the case of the *footbridge* (increased activity in the medial prefrontal cortex, including parts of the VMPFC), but he cannot assume from the start that, in the *switch* case (increased activity in the DLPFC), the utilitarian answer is *the right one*. He needs arguments to establish that, but he did not provide a single one. Besides, his criticism of Kant's ethics as based on "people's *rights*" is simply flawed (Greene, 2013, 115). Kant's ethics is based on *duties*, not on rights. I will return to this point below.

consequentialist approach in normative ethics. From John Stuart Mill onwards, many sophisticated forms of utilitarianism show that the best thing do to is to protect rights. Famously, in his last chapter of *Utilitarianism*, Mill shows the internal connection between justice and utility by arguing that rights, including *moral* ones, are justified and, therefore, protected under the supreme principle of morality. Thus, *pace* Greene and other naturalistic accounts of morality, rights and duties are *not* weapons of choice that allow us to present our feelings as nonnegotiable facts. As we will see, to respect a person is to defer to her rights, for instance, to her intrinsic autonomy. Recognizing a person's basic right to be free is what morality itself demands, and without liberty there is no morality. Therefore, Greene seems mistaken when he argues that "By appealing to rights, we excuse ourselves from the hard work of providing real, non-question-begging justifications for what we want." (2013, 304.) As we will see, a system of intrinsic rights can be justified by an appeal to the first principle of ethics; therefore, contrary to what the author of *Moral Tribes* held, they have nothing to do with feelings or emotions. To be a person just *is* to have rights and duties. Thus, it is not difficult to answer the question "Who has which rights?" Besides, Geene's attempt to transform utilitarianism into "deep pragmatism" (do *whatever works best*!) falls short of finding the first ethical principle. Once again, *neuro*ethics fails to provide a sound normative approach to deal with the moral problems we face nowadays, especially in doing neuroscience and applying it. From a care ethics perspective, Greene's formalistic principle is incapable of guiding moral actions.[36]Therefore, we must look for better foundations, and a conceptual analysis of both "care" and "respect" would lead us to a first principle in normative ethics, which will be presented in the last section of this chapter.

I would now like to differentiate between *general* and *especial* kinds of care to make sense also of the distinction between holistic bioethics and *special bioethics* or neuro*bioethics*. Let us, then, agree that *special* care is directed towards individuals such as parents, children, patients, close friends, etc. to whom we have certain close relationships that generate strong obligatory commitments and consequently specific actions. These are *special obligations* in our moral life and are, in some sense, agent-relative. Perhaps the most common case of special care is illustrated by the parent/child model, but clinical treatment is also a form of special care, which comes in many different degrees (intensive, primary, palliative etc.).

[36] Greene is simply mistaken about the groundlessness of rights discourses since even a utilitarian may, through the Greatest Happiness Principle, be able to provide a sound justificiation for rights (see, for instance, Brandt,1992; Railton, 2003). I will return to this point in the next section.

In this context, we may speak of *taking care of* one's safety, health, etc. Thus, there are many subspecies of special care, and I will certainly not be able to cover all its forms in this work. Now, special care relates mainly to non-autonomous individuals (perhaps, a teen such as Aysha), who are not agents in the strict sense, and other non-human animals as well. Note, however, that if A is a parent and B is not, then A has reasons for caring for a particular person that B does not. Consider what is called "Kangaroo Care": skin to skin contact between a parent and a baby. That is why parental care seems not to be, in some sense, agent-relative. In a clinical case, providing palliative care, especially for premature babies, is tied to specific professional roles. Thus, palliative care generates reasons for action which are in some sense agent-relative. On the other hand, everyone has reasons to hold that a baby must be cared for; in this sense, they are agent-neutral.

General care or *Cura* (caring about; not taking care of) is an attitude of concern which may include not only persons but the environment and all living creatures, and even material objects. Some ethicists, for example Noddings, have already applied care theory to non-human entities. She argued, in chapter 7 of *Caring*, that one may care for animals, plants, things and ideals. *Cura* is, then, a general attitude towards the world, which does not generate strong, direct and perfect obligations regarding particular individuals. Thus, one can say that the moral principle of general beneficence is related to *Cura*, but, more importantly, that the principle of non-maleficence is a universal foundation of such an attitude. No one is ever justified in gratuitously harming people, animals, the environment, etc. As can be seen, then, perhaps the most basic meaning of "care" simply implies the obligation to refrain from causing harms.

It is crucial, then, to recognize that there are different kinds of care and most important for the purposes of this work is to differentiate between moral and non-moral caring. A person may, for instance take care of her books in the library. This means among other things that she may protect them from damage, but that she is not worried about their well-being. This form of caring has no moral significance, since, as we have seen, caring has a special dimension when it instantiates an intrinsic valuation. Thus, not all kinds of care relate to the well-being of sentient beings. I will not concern myself with these types of care here. Moreover, different kinds of care sometimes may be provided only by special agents, for example, highly specialized nursing care for *the brain* not forgetting the person as a whole. In some sense, then, care presupposes a special kind of agent-relativity. It requires cutting-edge scientific knowledge and development through training in specialized skills. Thus, not everyone is required to care for an extremely vulnerable baby in a neonatal facility. What we need to ask then is the specific question most care ethicists are mainly concerned with: under which conditions does a person generally care for vulnerable being sin a respectful manner? Before presenting an analysis of this, I would like to reconstruct very briefly some recent discussions concerning care theory.

As was pointed out by Laura Cabrera (2017, 440), care ethics is an important normative framework for discussing neuroethics, for instance, at the intersection of the brain and mental health and the environment, especially in its relational aspects. Now, in recent years, care has received a great deal of scientific and philosophical attention. It started with Carol Gilligan's psychological studies of moral development in the constructivist Piagetian-Kohlbergian paradigm (which divides moral development into levels going from pre-conventional –based on authority, emotions, virtues etc.– to post-conventional –based on principles–) and her discovery of a "different voice". Now, perhaps against Gilligan's own intentions, which, as we will see, point to *complementary* voices, some authors thought it possible to explain all moral life from a caring perspective. For instance, this feminine moral voice was further investigated under Noddings' idea of "centuries of moral experience more typical of woman than men". One consequence of Gilligan's studies was, then, to divide ethics into two parties: on the one hand, there are those defending a morality of universal principles and rights, stressing equality and fairness and explaining the moral life as centered on equal respect among persons, thus expressing a rational, supposedly male, view; on the other hand, there are those pointing out that morality has to do with the recognition of differences in need, with personal responsibility to close relationships and with moral sentiments such as compassion, a supposedly female view. This division was not Gilligan's own view, but unfortunately it became commonplace in contemporary ethics.

I would like then to emphasize the point that there are many varieties of care ethics. For the purpose of distinguishing them, I will follow Lindemann's characterization of both an ethics of care and its distinctiveness from a feminist care ethics. According to her (2006, 92), the general features of an ethics of care are: (i) the centrality of close relationships; (ii) the engagement with another's will and; (iii) the attention paid to particulars. Virginia Held, (2006, 10-13) who, in my view, best developed this approach philosophically, adds some more features: an ethics of care values emotion rather than rejects it (and does not value more abstract reasoning leading to impartiality) and also reconceptualizes the private/public distinction leading to a more realistic conception of the person against the predominant individualistic theories of justice. Now, these features may or not lead to a particularistic approach to moral phenomena. Some care ethicists think that there is no way to care for everyone's well-being, that care is restricted to those around us –our family, our friends, perhaps the citizens of our state– but not all human beings.

I believe we should reject a particularist approach to the ethics of care, especially if we, as Held and Lindemann seem to do, want to keep a feminist basic assumption, namely that *there is no morally justifiable hierarchy of gender*. *A* CS-Morality is an egalitarian and a universalist one and this implies that *any* discrimination based on class, gender, ethnic, religious, cultural, nationality or other *secondary* features of a human agent is philosophically ungrounded. Thus, if we abstract the irrelevant features of any single human individual, we will reach a better understanding of the moral *person*, which allows us to achieve the aims of a feminist ethics of care. Therefore, an ethics of care is universalist, and there is a sense in which *a* CS-Morality does prescribe caring for strangers and not only individuals in caring *relations*, such as in the case of not polluting the environment, which may affect everyone's life; otherwise, there is no way of, *pace* some feminists and care theorists, criticizing patriarchalism, machismo and many other discriminations women face around the world.

The above features of care ethics may, however, be seen in a different light. They are not *per se* incompatible with general or even universal norms such as "first, do no harm", which apply to every single moral agent. It does not matter whether one lives in the US or in Brazil; one is never justified in producing only harm or more harms than benefits to Aysha. All we need to do to recognize this point is present a plausible account of moral reasoning as exemplified in a practical syllogism, for instance, by using a universal principle as the major premise, a minor rule to pay attention to the particulars, and the prescription that follows as the conclusion. Thus, in this sense, the present book is not, strictly speaking, a work in the ethics of care, if such an ethics is particularist, despite having many points in common. Moreover, I do not think that we can take all the moral elements out of care; for example, the obligation to *respect* negative rights cannot be justified as a form of care. That is why I will keep these two notions, namely care and respect, distinct, despite the fact that I will argue that they form a coherent whole, *limiting* and, at the same time, *complementing* each other.

An ethics of care, as indeed any ethical theory, must be aware of the problem of exploitation (caring jobs are less well-paid and are normally undertaken by women), the problem of integrity (the caregiver sacrificing her life's projects to care for others) and the problem of obliviousness to social justice (gender inequalities). This leads perhaps to a distinct *feminist* approach to the ethics of care, the so-called "second wave" of care ethics.

One problem here, however, isto define clearly "feminism" and to establish what is distinctive about this approach since there are many versions of feminism.[37] There is no doubt that a feminist care ethics takes seriously the political implications of caring-functions such as mothering or nursing, and social problems such as economic exploitation and domestic violence. This, however, depends on assuming an egalitarian morality, such as *a* CS-Morality, in order to be able to criticize these social pathologies leading to *emancipation,* which is feminism's main ideal. It is crucial to recognize that actions motivated by power usually lead to harm, from emotional and psychological abuse to physical violence. Moreover, most forms of power are in direct opposition to morality conceived as a way of intrinsically valuing an individual. Thus, this work is also not a feminist one in this sense, despite the fact that I strongly believe in the equality of persons irrespective of their sexual or gender orientations: I am at this point not concerned with power-relations, which are mainly political issues, but with what intrinsically valuing persons amounts to. Besides, there are forms and forms of exercising power, some legitimate, some not. Intrinsically valuing someone stands in opposition to the exercise of *illegitimate power*, that is, the use of force, violence, etc. Before arguing for this conclusion, let me analyze care in a more detailed way.

One of the first conditions constitutive of caring for, not only in the human case, seems then to be the capacity for sympathizing, that is, of *sympathetic concern.* As Darwin showed in *The Descent of Man* (2006), following Hume (sympathy) and Smith ("empathy"), this is a natural gift of any social creature, not just humans, and is necessary for survival. Sympathetic concern is an interspecies phenomenon, and many non-human animals exhibit it towards humans, so reciprocity seems to demand that we show it to them too. Sympathy moves us towards others. But sympathy is not enough and may even lead to wrongdoing, as many feelings and emotions sometimes do. One must also *know-how* to preserve or to increase the well-being of a vulnerable individual in effective ways. Thus, natural care becomes cultural, and if care is to have a moral connotation, then it *must* be practiced for the sake of those who need it only. There is no doubt, however, that caring involves, as has been pointed out by care ethicists and most contemporary feminist thinkers, sympathizing with individuals

---

[37] In Lindemann's own words: "Although feminists disagree about this, my own view is that feminism isn't –at least not directly– about equality, and it isn't about women, and it isn't about difference. *It's about power.*" (2006 p.9; italics added.) One great concern of most neuroethicists is the possibility *of controlling* the mind, but how this is something peculiar in terms of power relations is unclear. I will discuss this point in the next chapter.

(human beings or other non-human animals), paying attention to their basic necessities and positively answering them in ways that benefit and increase *their* well-being.

Moral caring for is directed at the *well-being* or welfare of a sentient being. This is its proper object. Thus, in order to clarify this condition, it is necessary to ask what the well-being of a vulnerable being comprises. For methodological reasons, I will here limit the analysis to human beings only, especially in neurobioethical contexts where a patient is at the same time a subject of experimental research. Now, to be coherent with agnosticism and value pluralism plus the project of *a* CS-Morality, we may not expect to answer this question by pointing to a single property of well-being (for instance, virtue or pleasantness) valid to all humans, but we need to provide a *mixed theory* of well-being. That is to say, some elements will, in some sense, be agent-relative (e.g., the sense of achievement of the life plan of an individual) and others will be agent-neutral (for instance, improving her health). Thus, well-being is here taken to be a complex concept: a set of different ingredients, including health, but not restricted to it. The one caring will only be successful in enhancing the well-being of the cared for by taking into consideration what the vulnerable being herself wants regarding what is valuable in her personal life, and, at the same time, fostering in the best way possible the agent-neutral elements of welfare; for example, satisfying the basic necessities everyone has. If this is not the case, then it is not possible to integrate care and respect and we will arrive at either paternalism or indifference.

Another condition of taking care of relates to care's proper moral dimension. That is to say, caring for someone vulnerable is best seen as *intrinsically valuing* that individual. To further discuss the example presented above (supposing for instance that Aysha has cognitive impairments), it is clear that a health professional seeks to benefit the patient, and that means, in the clinical context, *curing* her, restoring her health by embarking on a course of healing treatment. If a health professional really cares for a patient, she would not just consider whether she should satisfy her actual wishes (to increase treatment even if pointless), but she would think about what is good for *the patient herself*, that is, for *her* welfare. Thus, knowing-how to cure the patient is essential, as it is *knowing-how* to value her intrinsically. The one caring must foster the well-being of the cared for because this is good for *her* own sake. There is no real care if the one caring benefits the cared for out of selfish or self-interested reasons only. In this sense, care is always caring *for* someone, and this is only possible if it goes along with an intrinsic valuation. *A* CS-Morality requires that a person cares for a vulnerable being because this is good for her own sake. In other words, caring is intrinsically valuing a vulnerable individual because it is good for her, because it fosters *her* well-being.

To have one's well-being improved, out of sympathy, and for one's *own* sake, is what our analysis reveals moral caring for is all about. Caring for is, in this sense, a response to fundamental human needs such as breathing, drinking unpolluted water, and having food. As such, it is universally required; that is, all humans owe their existence to care. It may well also be true for some non-human animals. Caring for means improving the welfare of a vulnerable individual, and part of this is satisfying her basic needs, but there is also the accomplishment of one's own projects etc. This is not only related to one particular lifestyle but must also be compatible with all reasonable ones. A vulnerable individual's welfare cannot be related to acting virtuously. Moreover, we have the problem of divergent moralities with different sets of virtues: what is virtuous for a Christian (humility) may sound like a character deficiency for an Aristotelian or another virtue ethicist. Therefore, a CS-Morality should make room for divergences in beliefs and values. This is, as we will see in the next section, what respect is all about.

Care cannot be considered just a virtue among others, as some ethicists hold, nor can it be reduced to a form of virtue ethics. Despite the fact that we could accept a *formal* criterion to distinguish right from wrong actions, considering what a virtuous person would do in the circumstances as well as the thesis that virtues are intrinsically valuable, it does not follow that we need to abandon modernity and revive a form of ancient ethics. Thus, MacIntyre's appeal (1994) to traditionalism is philosophically unsustainable. Moreover, Kant's criticism right at the beginning of the *GMM* (4: 394) of *unprincipled* virtues is very convincing. Once again, we can realize why neuroscience cannot deliver us a sound normative ethics. That is to say, some neuroscientists clearly follow virtue ethics in defining moral judgment in terms of character traits.[38]The modern notion of morality is a point of no return in doing ethical theory.

Having presented an examination of "care" and discussed some varieties of care ethics, I would now like to consider the main contributions care thinkers could bring to (neuro)bioethics. It seems clear that caring for people with brain problems or people with mental disorders such as depression, schizophrenia, etc. could be seen as a fertile domain for this ethical approach. To understand what the concerns might be, we could go

---

[38] See Takahaski *et al.* Neural Correlates of Human Virtue Judgement. *Cereb Cortex*, 2008, 18. pp.1886-1891. Once again, whether a deontological, consequentialist or virtue approach in normative ethics is best suited for neuro*ethics* cannot be established by *neuro*ethics.

back to some questions posed by the O3, especially questions 4 and 5, namely: how is "care" constituted when it is delivered via an algorithm, or a robot and how should mental health and well-being apps be regulated? The answers to these questions depend, obviously, on how the robot or app is programmed. In my previous work on care delivered by artificial agents, I used the experiment of a *Person-o-Matic* machine to discuss the best caring robot, that is, a droid or a humanoid robot.[39] Thus, if, on the one hand, the droid is programmed with cutting-edge medical knowledge, has excellent caring skills, etc., but always does what *it* thinks –paternalistically– is best for you, and, on the other hand, the humanoid robot has the same knowledge and skills, but it is sensitive and open to your needs and wishes and respects your rights –including your right to self-determination– then I would prefer a *caring respectful* robot and not a mere robot caregiver. That is to say, it must be programmed to deliver *respectful care* or *caring respect* and regulated accordingly. Since we still need to discuss the concept of "respect" in order to formulate the notion of *caring* respect, I will return to this point later in this chapter and try to answer the other O3 questions as well.

To finish this section, it is necessary to emphasize that no person is in a complete state of non-vulnerability, not even human adults. Moreover, a human person may return to a state of vulnerability through accident or illness etc. or through ageing. Thus, mutual care is always required. Some forms of care must also be enforced by law and this goes under the label of "political care," which means the kind of care everyone needs to become a person. For instance, heathcare, educational care, security care etc. are essential for all of us. But most humans do not live in a state of deep vulnerability: the majority of us are adults and, so to speak, in good shape. This is to say, most of the time we are not ill, disabled or in a fragile condition (too young or too old). Consequently, we must take care of ourselves and respect others who are doing the same according to *their* worldview, *their* project of life, *their* conception of living well etc. Respect for persons becomes a central tenet of the moral life. I will, then, focus now on the other pole of *a* CS-Morality, namely reciprocal respect.

---

[39] Cf. Dall'Agnol, D. *Care and Respect in Bioethics*. Newcastle: Cambridge Scholars, 2016. p. 149. If we regard care as related to the person's well-being as a whole, then caring for the vulnerable includes caring for her brain and mental faculties too. The O3 Consortium asks whether there are any special concerns about care delivery in the context of mental health and well-being. Apparently, nothing in neuroscience challenges medical *ethics* with something completely new, for instance, when we treat mental disorders. I will discuss this point in detail in the last chapter.

2.2 – Respect for persons

As I said above, the main goal of this chapter is to present some of the main tenets of *a* moral system capable of integrating care and respect, two expressions of *knowing-how* to *intrinsically value* a vulnerable individual or a person, into a coherent whole. In the previous section, I made explicit the main ingredients of *taking care of* a vulnerable being. In the present part, I will do the same for the concept of *respect* to prepare the terrain for analyzing, in the next section, under which conditions we can say that a person *knows-how* to respect, in a caring manner, another person (e.g. Aysha if she is person).

To start with, I would like to discuss the concept of personhood and ask what "person" means after all. An answer to this question will then help to clarify the normative framework needed for neurobioethics.[40]At this point, then, it is crucial to bear in mind one of the middle level principles stated in the *Belmont Report*: respect for *persons* and not just respect for *autonomy*. Moreover, since we are looking for some illumination from neuroscience here, I would like to evaluate whether it has something to say on this issue.

Now, "what is a person?" is a conceptual, not an empirical, question. This issue must be crystal clear at this point: defining a concept comes *prior* to looking for what instantiates it; for example, before asking whether Pluto is a planet or not, we need to have a clear conception of "planet". The same applies to ethical concepts. That is to say, before deciding whether a baby or a teenager or a coma patient is a person, we need to clarify what "person" means. Does it refer to any member of the species *Homo sapiens* or just to individuals who happen to be agents as is the common use in a forensic context to hold people accountable?

Some neuroethicists believe we can define personhood in neuroscientific terms. According to Martha J. Farah, it was "The promise of a definition of personhood, anchored in the functioning of a physical,

---

[40] As we have already seen, to avoid the mereological fallacy (the fallacy of ascribing to a part predicates that apply only to a whole and making afterwards invalid reasonings), Bennet and Hacker proposed considering "the human being as a whole," that is, as "a psychophysical unity." I am very sympathetic to this approach to personhood, but we should perhaps consider other dimensions as well, as some neuroethicists do, taking persons as *bio-psycho-spiritual* beings (Grosso 2013, p.55f.) or rather biopsychosocial entities (including the ethical in the social). These approaches have interesting practical implications, for instance in clinical neuroethics, leading to a person-based healthcare system. I will develop to this point in the last chapter.

objectively observable system has led many bioethicists to neuroscience." (2010, 296) I do not believe, however, that neuroscience can give us a final definition of a person without committing the mereological fallacy, but let us investigate the arguments grounding this promise. Basically, it says that a set of psychological traits such as intelligence, rationality, self-awareness, cognition about the future, linguistic communication, consciousness, etc. are normally attributed to a person. Since these mental states can be established in terms of the brain's *functions*, the conclusion that follows is that personhood is a function of the brain. This is a clear example of how a reductionist account works. Before critically discussing it, I would like to reconstruct some of the ethical implications of such an account.

In their work "Personhood: An Illusion Rooted in Brain Function?" Martha J. Farah and Andrea S. Heberlein argued that personhood is in fact an illusion. According to them (2010, 320):

> Personhood is a foundational concept in ethics, yet defining criteria have been elusive. Here we explore the possibility that personhood has been so hard to pin down because it is an illusion. According to this view, "persons" does not correspond with a category of objects in the world. Rather, it is an illusory concept that our brains have evolved to develop innately and project onto the world whenever triggered by stimulus features such as a human-like face, body, or contingent patterns of behavior.

Granted, *persons* are not natural *objects* in the world like plants, but should we not look for personhood elsewhere, not using neuroimaging but a more suitable methodological instrument, namely conceptual analysis, which must be carried out *prior* to reducing persons to physical entities only?

Apart from the reductionistic assumption (a whole being to one of its parts, the brain), the definition of "person" in neuroscientific terms seems to miss the *moral* dimension completely. That is to say, a person is basically an agent who is a *rights' holder* and a *bearer of obligations*, so she cannot be reduced to her mental or physical states. Even if one uses a naturalist conception of person, for instance simply identifying it with a member of the species *Homo sapiens*, we would still need to discriminate agents from non-agents for ethical-juridical purposes.

Consider Farah & Heberlin's claim that neuroscience suggests the existence of a separate system for representing persons and a person network that is automatic and innate. They present as evidence the fact that newborns within 30 minutes of birth show a greater tendency to track moving facelike patterns. I do not question that, but I would like to ask what this is supposed to show. Does it prove that persons are just agents with a human face? Is that sufficient, for instance, for the juridical role of assigning actions to agents because they did not act as was morally required? Is a social institution not a person? Is a bonobo not a person? Is an autonomous robot not a person? It seems clear that we are dealing with a conceptual question, not an empirical one. The conclusion should be that neuroscience is incapable of defining personhood because it takes into consideration only natural objects. It has misleading nihilistic implications.

Strange as it may seem, then, it appears that *the main challenge* from the neurosciences is related to the existence of ethics itself. There is a widespread tendency to argue that there is no free will, that personhood is an illusion, etc. In this context, I would briefly like to discuss Farah's and Heberlein's scientificist approach to neuroethics and its nihilistic implications. They are aware of this consequence and explicitly defend it, since their conclusion is the following:

> The result of this analysis could be considered *nihilistic*. It does undercut ethical systems based on personhood and in particular suggests that difficult ethical issues should not be approached with the strategy of determining whether or not the parties involved are persons. If personhood is not really in the world, then there is no fact of the matter concerning the status of a given being as a person or not, and there is no point to the philosophical or bioethical program of seeking objective criteria for personhood more generally because there are none. (Farah and Heberlein 2010, 334; italics added)

Strangely enough, however, the nihilistic implications apply only to deontological theories based on personhood (Kantian ethics based on respect, rights-based theories etc.), but not to utilitarianism. Furthermore, their final proposal is unjustified since they argue for a shift to a more utilitarian approach in ethics while continuing to use the concept of personhood in everyday moral life. This is clearly a flawed ethical theory based on scientistic assumptions. It may be true that "neuroscience could reduce us to machines" (Farah 2010, 8), but neurobio*ethics* is here precisely to prevent that by enforcing the moral imperative: Do not use persons! Neurobio*ethics* seeks to protect and enhance personhood, not abolish it.

The concept of personhood is an ethical, not a natural one. It is necessary in law and elsewhere to make sense of many of our intersubjective practices. Agency, which is a *natural* property of human and some non-human individuals, is a necessary condition, but not a sufficient one. To be a person, one needs to have an ethical property recognized: her rights and obligations. We may realize this if we look at what happens when they are denied: in slavery, de-personalization is precisely not recognizing the moral rights of a human being for instance to her liberty. Thus, the argument I would like to present here to show that personhood is a necessary precondition for accountability and, therefore, not just an illusion, is the following:

P1: If there were persons, then we would not be able to correctly attribute rights and responsibilities to entities capable of acting.

P2: We do attribute rights and responsibilities to entities capable of acting and hold them accountable for their deeds.

Therefore: there are persons.

If this argument is sound (valid and correct), then personhood cannot just be an illusion or a fiction. It is a necessary condition not only to attribute actions to agents, but, most importantly, rights and/or obligations. It follows, then, that Farah and Heberlien do not have a sound ground to establish utilitarianism against a rights-based normative ethics. I will return to their account of personhood in the next chapter while discussing other *nihilistic* implications of doing *neuro*ethics from the narrow perspective of the neuroscience of morality.

Given the argument just presented, we may now proceed to the analysis of another fundamental material tenet of *a* CS-Morality, namely respect for persons. For this reason, I will sort out the ingredients of "respect" and start to explore some of its practical implications. As we have seen, care is a condition for all humans to become persons, that is, autonomous beings. Now, given agnostic pluralism, persons must learn *how* to respect each other's beliefs and values even if they are opposing and perhaps incompatible. This does not mean that respect is just a by-product of care as some care theorists have argued. On the contrary, to avoid paternalism we need to recognize that respect *limits* care and that there are rights which cannot be justified by care, for instance, the right to negative freedom. This is one of the main limitations of an ethics based purely on care. Thus, I will argue that respect is another fundamental ingredient of *a* CS-Morality, which also plays a fundamental role in our moral life, for instance, in protecting a person's rights. Moreover, we need to sort out what rights a person has, for example, to be cared for, to privacy, etc.

As for care ethics, there are many varieties of an ethics based on universal respect. The most wellknown is inspired by Kant's idea of rational beings as ends in themselves. The fundamental assumption is that a rational being has a kind of absolute value, namely *dignity*, which cannot be measured in quantitative terms, that is, it cannot be reduced to price. It is for this reason that it is said that money cannot buy a person. The basic idea is that a person is an end in herself and must be treated as such. Dignity gives rise to respect, that is, forms of action and attitudes which are not manipulative in the sense of, for example, enslaving persons, deceiving them and so on. The Universal Declaration of Human Rights (UDHR) seems to rely on this special value. Now, this concept of "dignity" is, however, based on a particular worldview related to a Judeo-Christian morality, namely on the metaphysical assumption that humans were created in God's image. Kant was well aware of that, since, despite claiming to have established a non-theological basis for morality, he clearly postulated the traditional metaphysical dogmas such as the immortality of the soul as a condition for accomplishing the supreme good (virtue and happiness united in an afterlife). Kant's ethics, then, does not appeal to everyone anymore, and, consequently, it cannot form the basis of a truly universal morality such as *a* CS-Morality needs to be. It may though be a fundamental value for that particular moral system, and persons belonging to it are entitled to believe and act accordingly. I think that a similar metaphysical assumption is behind Rawls' notion of respect for persons: each person possesses an inviolability founded on justice that even the welfare of society as a whole cannot override (Rawls 1999, 3). This is clearly an overstatement. Thus, *a* CS-Morality cannot depend on it, and other moral systems are not obligated to incorporate it. This becomes clearer if we bear in mind that it is possible to naturalize the concept of dignity, defining it in terms of the quality of life a person has. For example, differently from Kant, other philosophers postulate an "external" notion of dignity as social recognition of a person's role in society. Thus, there is no way to solve this semantic point, except by recalling agnosticism in metaphysics. If we are to keep a principle such as *respect for persons*, it must have no metaphysical assumptions. For *a* CS-Morality, all that is needed is a conception of a *person as a rule-following entity,* that is, as an autonomous being (agent) who is, at the same time, a rights' holder and a bearer of obligations. All human beings, at least dispositionally, are persons. Some non-human animals are too, and in the near future artificial agents may also have their personhood recognized.

What is then crucial is to identify the proper object of respect in order to avoid these metaphysical problems. Now, according to some recent ethicists, the proper object of moral respect is the person's rights. This was clearly emphasized by the German philosopher Ernst Tugendhat (among others), who is perhaps best-known in Anglophone philosophy for his project of a formal semantics. I believe Tugendhat is right about the main contents of Kantian ethics, and I have already analyzed his contributions to an ethics of universal respect, but I would like briefly to sum them up here.

According to Tugendhat's first approach to ethics back in the 1980s saying that a moral system is justified means basically three things: (i) it corresponds to everyone's empirical interests; (ii) it is equally good;

(iii) it is universally good (1988, 9).[41] We could adopt these assumptions for *a* CS-Morality. This view about the foundations of a moral system does not compromise faced either with a superior truth (for example, a metaphysical or a theological one) or with any assumption about pure "Reason" (with capital R) as an infallible human faculty capable of establishing the supreme principle of morality once and for all, as Kant claimed. It also does not make any assumption about what human beings are for, or about the essence of mankind, like some Aristotelians seem to believe is necessary in order to establish the foundations of morality. All is needed is just a Wittgensteinian assumption of sharing a lifeform, which could, by the way, be found in Aristotle (what is good for humans, not the good in itself) and Kant (right for rational, but finite beings). Finally, it does not commit to the view that the particular *ethos* of a specific community is the only criterion for the right and the good, that is, the intrinsically valuable.

Now, in *Vorlesungen über Ethik*, Tugendhat (1994) engaged in a reformulation of Kant's Categorical Imperative to overcome some weaknesses of the contractual model, namely that it is incapable of grounding moral equality, proper motivation etc. To avoid such difficulties, one important alternative is to reform Kant's ethics in terms of respect for persons as bearers of rights and/or obligations. As it is well known, one of Kant's formulae of the Categorical Imperative is this: "Act in such a way that you always treat humanity, whether in your own person or in the person of any other, never simply as a means, but always at the same time as an end." (GMM 4: 429) But, according to Tugendhat, there is no clear distinction between treating a person as a means or as a *mere* means. Kant's examples seem flawed; for example, pre-marital sexual intercourse is not always instrumental and indeed rape may happen within a marriage. Now, Tugendhat argues that we need to reformulate Kant's supreme principle of morality in the updated vocabulary of rights and obligations. His principle is, "Act (toward everyone) as you, from the perspective of any person, would want everyone to act."[42] This principle is capable of justifying

[41] I coined the label "protocontractualism" to denote this way of analyzing the foundations of a moral system. What is its main proposition? It is this: one has reasons to accept a moral system if one can justify in front of others that they, like oneself, have reasons (motives) to accept and submit themselves to it. In this way, a moral system is justified if it is good, that is, if it corresponds to the interest of a person being equally and universally acceptable. It provides, however, too weak a justification for *a* CS-Morality as we will see soon.

[42] "handle so (allengegenüber) wie du aus der Perspektiveeinerbeliebigen Person wollenwürdest, dassallehandeln." (Tugendhat 1994, p.83) Thanks to Professor Rauscher for helping me with the translation from German into English.

particular rules and virtues as well. As we will see in the next section, however, this can perhaps be put in Parfitian terms, namely respect for persons could be universally willable. Now, according to Tugendhat, to respect a person means basically to defer to her rights. By respecting persons, we respect all sorts of rights and agree to fulfil the corresponding obligations.

I would like to point out now that, more recently, Tugendhat has become disillusioned with this Kantian analysis of a morality of universal respect and has gone back to his previous model. However, I deplore Tugendhat's return to ethical (proto)contratualism. The main reason for this being that a principle of equality or the idea of persons as autonomous agents is always a necessary presupposition in any contractualist theory including Rawls' theory of justice as fairness. That is why Tugendhat's contractualism or other Rawlsian views such as Engelhardt's autonomism or Veath's triple contractualist model in bioethics need to be based on a stronger foundation, such as the one provided by *a first principle of ethics* for *a* CS-Morality, which assumes these ideas as necessary to make pluralism reasonable. The fundamental ethical principle could be considered, in Wittgensteinian terms, a *hinge-proposition*, which makes possible contingent contracts, but the real basic agreement is in sharing our lifeform (PI §241). I will present such a first principle as an ethical hinge-proposition in the next section.

The need for universal respect has been correctly emphasized by many other contemporary Kantian ethicists. For instance, inspired by Kant's distinction between *reverentia* (respect for persons) and *observantia* (respect for the moral law), Darwall distinguishes between appraisal respect and recognition respect. Now, according to him, "The esteem we call 'respect' –henceforth *appraisal respect*– is an assessment of someone's conduct or character or of something that somehow involves these. Appraisal respect for someone as a person is moral esteem: the approbation for her as a moral agent." (2006, 122) Appraisal respect depends on the agent's actions and therefore on merit. We respect perhaps saints and heroes in this sense. Now, "By contrast, the respect we can demand as persons regardless of our merit is no form of esteem at all. ... The object is recognition respect is not excellence or merit; it is dignity or authority," (Darwall 2006, 122-3). The latter is the recognition of one's personhood and generates agent-relative reasons for actions (in the positional sense). But, in the non-positional sense, it generates also agent-neutral reasons for action. Clearly, then, there are different *kinds of respect*. One may respect property; one can be respectful of others by being polite, etc. But the most important *moral* notion is recognition respect, which cannot, however, be based on a metaphysical notion of dignity. We may then have the same reasons to reject this presupposition of recognition respect as we did for Kant's idea of dignity. Moreover, Kant's most basic idea is that we must respect the moral law and that, by doing so, we will respect persons.

Having reconstructed some discussions in contemporary ethics on the idea of respect for persons, I am now in a better position to present a conceptual examination of "respect." In order to do so, it is important to recall the two main results of the previous chapter that applied to care as well. First, there is the epistemic condition; that is, one needs to *know-how* to respect a person, for instance, by not infringing on or violating her rights. Second, to be a full moral attitude, respect must exhibit an *intrinsic valuation*. I will now spell out these conditions in more detail.

First of all, it seems clear that an individual must be *recognized* as such, that is, as a person. As human history shows us, slavery was only possible because people did not recognize, for example, pre-Columbian indigenous peoples or Africans as persons. However, as the terminological origin of the word "respect" (from Latin, *re-spectare*) makes clear, to respect means to *look back*, to look again in order to *recognize* them as persons. Thus, the word "*re*-cognize" keeps this feature of the term. That is to say, respecting a person requires *knowing-how* to recognize an individual as an agent, that is, as a bearer of rights and responsibilities. To give another example: to respect a patient/subject of neuroscientific research is to look at that individual again and consider her as a *person* and not only as a patient, that is, as capable of deciding whether or not she needs more care. As a person, the patient has the right to decide what to do in the circumstances. Consequently, to recognize a person *qua* person is a basic condition to give her what she is entitled to as a moral agent equal to everyone else.

Second, a person must be regarded as a rights' holder, but at the same time, a bearer of obligations. Most present-day declarations following the UDHR overemphasize the rights of individuals and the obligations of states. Thus, some individuals have too many expectations about rights and no idea about their obligations. Now, there is no doubt that as a person everyone is entitled, for instance, to lead the life one chooses, but this is granted only if it generates an obligation for everyone else to respect the choices of every person. Here, pluralism, as discussed previously, makes plain sense: a person has the right to choose not only to which worldview she wants to belong and to enforce it, but what kind of lifestyle she prefers: a life of pleasures or a life of philosophical thinking or a life of economic activities or a life of artistic enjoyment or a life of political realizations or a life of religious devotion and so on and so forth. All are meaningful and, consequently, worth living. Because of this diversity of lifestyles and the plurality of intrinsic goods, it is natural to disagree and have divergent opinions on how to behave in particular circumstances. In all styles of life, however, respect must be incorporated. Every person, regardless of her way of life, beliefs, etc. must give respect to those who think and live differently, and, in turn, may expect respect, or better, *extract* respect from others. Thus, reciprocal respect is a fundamental condition for pacific co-existence and many forms of cooperation (economic, scientific, cultural, etc.).

Finally, it seems clear that fulfilling one's obligations towards a person's rights is a condition for respecting her. One must defer to a person's rights because they are *her* rights, so an intrinsic valuing is always involved in the attitude of respecting. Of the correspondent obligations generated by these rights, some are personal obligations and some are public, that is, everyone's responsibility. If a teenager has the right to self-determination, then a professor or a school must fulfil her obligations and give her the best possible educational care. Many rights, however, generate obligations not to particular agents, but to the community as a whole. Thus, *a* CS-Morality provides the rationale for the state to be the public institution responsible for enforcing the rights that are everyone's responsibility. As we will see, we can apply a principle based on the concepts being investigated here to politics, for example, as Dworkin does (1977) when he argues that "equal concern and respect" provides legitimacy to government. I will return to this point later.

As I pointed out above, there are many kinds of respect, and they may have only family resemblances. Thus, the above analysis does not lead to a single use of the concept of "respect." What it does though is lay down a rule for the use of the expression *respect for persons* in the moral sense necessary to build up *a* CS-Morality. But we may here think of the concept of a reverential attitude as a kind of respect, for instance, for life as a whole. I have, based on Dworkin's argument (1993) that bioethical problems must be faced using the notion of the intrinsic value of life, proposed the following middle level principle for ecoethics and zooethics: *revere life's inherent worth*. As many philosophers have argued, life as a whole, independently of whether it is the result of divine intervention or the result of natural investment, must be respected. Perhaps the best word here to describe this attitude is *reverentia* for life. It may have only some resemblance to the concept of respect for persons, but it has many important applications in environmental and animal ethics.

We can now extract some practical implications of the above model. The complete specification of the principle of respect for persons will only be possible after sorting out, so to speak, a table of rights. One point, however, needs to be discussed here. If "having a right" means having a *subjective* claim (a person may decide to exercise it or not), then this implies that it does not always generate concrete obligations but may only make actions permissible. This may explain why some matters give rise to intractable and interminable discussions. For example, regarding the bioethical issue of the end of life, there is no consensus about whether voluntary euthanasia for the terminally ill is permissible: some value systems prohibit it; some allow it. It seems that there is no single, right answer here. Besides, both palliative care and assistance in dying might be seen as expressions of a caring and respectful attitude. Thus, it introduces some degree of *apparent* relativism. In fact, considering agnosticism and pluralism, it is clear that there is no unique and *final* answer to such questions. Specific approaches to this issue depend on particular worldviews or basic beliefs. Thus, *a* CS-Morality requires each person to decide by herself on this issue grounding her right to do so.

This brings us to one more question: "*Which* rights does the person have?" Granted, the person, as a moral entity, is distinct from all other things in the world: *it has rights and obligations, not price*. In this way, we must look for the rights a person has *qua* person. Inspired by Henry Shue's 1980 list of three basic rights (the trichotomy: security, subsistence and liberty), I would like to present a system of intrinsic rights of the person. Thus, my proposal is here to consider he following system of *intrinsic* moral rights as constitutive of personhood itself: (i) to a safe existence; (ii) to basic equalities and fairness; and (iii) to political and civil liberties. In the first group, there are fundamental rights such as to life (in the case of living agents), security from all kinds of harms, satisfaction of basic necessities, assistance from a healthcare system, etc. In the second, there are basic rights such as equality before the law, impartial judgements in fair trials, economic equity, etc. Last, but not least, there are fundamental rights constitutive of personhood itself such as basic liberties like freedom of movement, property ownership, the ability to vote for a government and to be voted for, etc. I cannot spell out the complete system of intrinsic rights here, but this list gives us a general idea of what it takes *to respect persons*. The already mentioned UDHR may be seen as an instantiation of such a system, despite the fact that it could be improved to incorporate new rights. Apart from these intrinsic rights, there are contingent rights according to people's differences, for instance, in roles, professions, etc. Now, for *a* CS-Morality based on universal respect, it is clear that rights and obligations are co-originary: any intrinsic right you have has a correspondent obligation toward other persons, but, again, to present the whole system of rights/obligations goes beyond the limits of this work.

To finish this section, then, I would like, having presented an examination of both care and respect, to say one more thing regarding their nature as moral attitudes. As I showed in the previous chapter, there are many bearers of intrinsic worth, including moral and non-moral ones. I would then like to re-emphasize the feature that distinguishes intrinsically valuing in the moral sense, namely caring and respecting: they provide reasons for action that *override* other forms of inherent worth, for instance, aesthetical ones. Thus, in *a* CS-Morality there are objective ways of establishing what counts as acting rightly, which must be equal for everyone, and personal ways of choosing how to live well. That is to say, *a* CS-Morality is a system based on wisdom, that is, on knowing-how to act rightly and to live well, for instance, respectfully caring or, what could turn out to be the same basic moral attitude, respecting in a caring manner. That is not to say that care and respect stand for the same attitude. On the one hand, respect limits care, preventing paternalism both on the individual and on the institutional or political level; on the other hand, the absence of care leads to indifference and individualism. Consequently, *care without respect is blind; respect without care is empty.* We have now the necessary ingredients to build up the concept of *caring respect* in the next section.

2.3 –The concept of caring respect

In the last two sections, I argued for *a* CS-Morality and spelled out some of its main contents. It seems worthwhile here to recall the main points of such a moral system. We arrived at the idea of *a* CS-Morality as the condition for making pluralism, derived from the conception of philosophy as a search for wisdom, reasonable, and therefore avoiding radical relativism. This moral system is best described not in terms of the common-sense morality or in terms of what is contingently common to all existing value systems (*the* morality), but as *a sharable* morality based on what is *common* to all of us. I sorted out the two main ingredients of such *a* CS-Morality, namely caring for the vulnerable and respecting persons and provided a conceptual examination of both "care" and "respect." I have not discussed in detail the political components of caring for the vulnerable, especially a solid education, a safety net of organizations and a fair healthcare system. I have also not examined all the material elements of respect for persons; that is, I have not spelled out a complete system of intrinsic rights and the institutions needed to enforce it. But I have at this point identified the main material ingredients (care and respect) of *a* CS-Morality. In this section, then, I will discuss ways of looking at care and respect as integrated into a coherent moral system, that is, as the two main components of *a* CS-Morality, which may be in *tension*, but can and must form a harmonized whole. To achieve this aim, I will present a first ethical principle which definitely overcomes the intuitionist basis of the predominant approach in (neuro)bioethics and a conceptual analysis of "caring respect."

Before attempting to show how care and respect stand in tension but are matching aspects of *a* CS-Morality, I would like to remove some of the psychological, political, and meta-ethical obstacles of such an enterprise. I would like to start with some misunderstandings produced by the so-called "ethics of care". As we have seen, this ethical approach resulted from Gilligan's studies in moral development, which, according to some feminist ethicists, pointed to two incompatible moralities: we should choose between an ethics of respect for rights *or* an ethics of care. But, as Gilligan herself argued, and this is usually forgotten, these fundamental moral notions are in fact two sides of the same coin. Thus, she provides another clear way of overcoming present day dichotomies in normative ethics. In Gilligan's own words:

> The morality of rights is predicated on equality and centered on the understanding of fairness, while the ethics of responsibility relies on the concept of equity, the recognition of differences in need. While the ethics of rights is a manifestation of equal respect, balancing the claims of other and self, the ethics of responsibility rests on an understanding that gives rise to compassion and care. Thus, the counterpoint of identity and intimacy that marks the time between childhood and adulthood is articulated through two moralities whose *complementarity* is the discovery of maturity. (Gilligan 1993, 165; italics added)

Most writers follow Gilligan's studies uncritically, forgetting that the opposition between care and respect is a matter of infancy or adolescence and that *moral maturity* requires their integration into a coherent whole. That is to say, any mature person must care *and* respect regardless of his/her gender. Therefore, it seems that respectful care or caring respect is the unifying core *a* CS-Morality from a mature psychological perspective.

This is perhaps the best place to point out also that it is possible to incorporate some of the main contributions of care ethics into a more comprehensive theory while avoiding some of the particularist assumptions of such an approach. As some ethicists have pointed out, one may start with the ethics of care, that is, with the assumption that the relationships among particular individuals are central. But, then, it may turn out that a deontological and a consequentialist ethics are *not* incompatible with the idea that we must give attention to the individual "… to the extent that it can be derived from equal concern and respect for all." (Darwall 1998, 225). I think that Darwall is right in arguing that a sound care ethics is not incompatible with a deontic perspective, despite the fact that *some* varieties of the ethics of care, in fact, are. Such particularist accounts, however, can be refuted by focusing on the *common* features of our lifeform. Once again, we can see here how the three main normative approaches may converge. The same result can also be achieved by arguing that care and respect can be integrated into a coherent complex concept, for instance, caring respect.

Since we are on the way to matching these two notions, which isolated may lead to either indifference and individualism (respect without care) or many forms of paternalism (care without respect), I would like to recall the different ways some divergences in normative *ethical theory* can be overcome. This attempt is not a new one. Many ethicists think that there is a way of overcoming the current dichotomies between some forms of deontology and consequentialism. We have different ways of doing so: i) by proposing norms for bioethics, the *Belmont Report* gives *prima facie* weight to both deontological principles (respect for persons and justice) and a teleological one (beneficence), a blend the so-called "four-principles approach" took further by adding non-maleficence; ii) Hare's attempt to integrate the alleged Kantian *form* of moral language (the prescriptivity and overridingness of moral judgments alongside their universalizability) with a utilitarian *content*, namely the satisfaction of preferences; iii) Railton's sophisticated form of consequentialism, which incorporates deontic notions such as respect into the set of intrinsic values to be promoted; iv) sophisticated deontological theories such as Rawls' theory of justice as fairness and Habermas's ethics of discourse, which are not anti-consequentialist at all despite giving priority to "right" over "good"; and v) a Wittgensteinian clarificatory ethics as proposed by Wisnewski, which holds that Kant's Categorical Imperative describes the workings of *practical rationality* and that the Principle of Utility describes the conditions for *flourishing*; finally (vi), I would also like to recall that I have proposed an adjustment to Parfit's Triple Theory, which is one of the most recent attempts to overcome the polarization between deontology and consequentialism, by incorporating the *formal* criterion for right action from virtue ethics. There is no space here to discuss all these options, but I will return to some soon. Consequently, there is no more room for orthodox, radicalized forms of normative theories today. As Parfit held (2013, 411), it seems really to be the case that we are all climbing the same mountain from different angles.

To avoid misunderstandings, I would now like to point out in more detail why *a* CS-Morality based on respect for persons is not necessarily full-blooded anti-consequentialist. That is to say, it is compatible with sophisticated forms of consequentialism. Consider, for instance, Railton's list (2003, 163) of intrinsically valuable things to be maximized: happiness, knowledge, purposeful activity, autonomy, solidarity, respect and beauty. Despite the fact that I would not, in an Aristotelian spirit, put happiness as a good among others, I do agree with Railton that the results being sought are complex; that is, they comprise many intrinsic values. Now, if this includes things like autonomy, *respect*, rights, fairness, etc., then there is no incompatibility with a moderate deontologist ethics as in a crude hedonist form of utilitarianism. Granted, even for classical utilitarians such as Bentham and Mill, there was the principle "everybody to count for one, nobody for more than one" in tension with the "greatest good of the greatest number." In formal terms, however, one could say that counting everybody for one, that is, giving persons due respect, brings the best consequences; that is, it is optimific. Of course, there might be occasions when a sophisticated consequentialist must trade off all these goods in order to be able to see what to do, but this seems not to be a sufficient reason for not adopting a pluralist form of consequentialism. As I have been arguing, there are different ways of overcoming the dichotomy between deontology and consequentialism towards a unified normative approach.

This is not to say, however, that any form of deontology is acceptable. I have already rejected many tenets of Kant's ethics (the rigorist assumptions of an absolute good will), and a similar thought needs to be applied to some of its reformulations. Consider here Habermas's discursive ethics. This is based on a *procedure* similar to Rawls' original position, namely on an idealized community of speakers, who, following some conditions that make possible communication (intelligibility, veracity/sincerity, normative correction and truth), would agree on fundamental norms for action. But Habermas (1990) assumes also some particular values; for instance, everyone must be equally capable of presenting arguments and must *respect* other ideas, etc. despite pretending to present a purely *procedural* way of legitimizing norms. Moreover, I think that Tugendhat's objection (1994, 161f.) to discourse ethics is still cogent, namely that consensus is the criterion neither for truth nor for right action. On the contrary, it is what is right that makes it possible to achieve some agreement. For example, it is not the democratic framework of the idealized community of speakers that justifies democracy, but it is the latter that provides some of the appeal of the former. Therefore, *pace* Habermas, there are fundamental values presupposed in discursive ethics that are not subject to any intersubjective discussion.

My own work in normative ethics goes in the same direction. We cannot passively stand on a division of the main theories in deontology, consequentialism and virtue ethics. Thus, to mention some basic assumptions of my attempt to overcome this "manualistic" state of affairs (known as "the textbook approach" as we encounter in many introductory books to bioethics), I have analyzed both "good" and "right" in terms of "value" making it possible to refute the dichotomy between deontologists and consequentialists. I have called this "the non-priority meta-ethical thesis." Moreover, I have proposed regarding both actions and their effects as *organic wholes*, allowing for sophisticated forms of moral deliberation, which avoids both extreme forms of deontology (e.g., Kant's ethics, intuitionism etc.) and full-blooded kinds of consequentialism (ethical egoism, hedonism, classical utilitarianism etc.), since they do not make sense of our most basic moral experiences. Furthermore, I have defended a first principle of normative ethics which subsumes the formal aspects of the main theories. To make it work, I have refused Kant's absolutist notion of good will and reformulated his theory as a form of rule-consequentialism. In the same spirit, I have refused the hedonistic assumptions of classical Utilitarianism and accepted axiological pluralism towards a sophisticated form of *rule*-consequentialism. This means that I have also to reject act-consequentialism. This can be done by showing that it has many problems, for instance, our fallibility in finding out all the time the best consequences of breaking a moral rule. Thus, we need to overcome some ethical orthodoxy to arrive at a new philosophical landscape.

Bearing all these points in mind, I have recently reworked Parfit's Triple Theory into the following metanorm here proposed as the first ethical principle (FEP) for *a* CS-Morality:[43]

> FEP: *Follow norms that prescribe* prima facie *right actions, but are also optimific, uniquely universally willable and would not be rejected by a virtuous person.*

Basically, I have, apart from the above-mentioned remarks for overcoming radical forms of both deontology and consequentialism, made two main changes to Parfit's Triple Theory: (i) I expressed the metaprinciple in *normative* terms giving it a clear action-guiding role; (ii) I incorporated the formal criterion from virtue ethics (after all, reasonableness can be seen as one particular character trait). This first principle needs no proof, since it is

[43] Parfit's original formula is this one: "an act is wrong just when such acts are disallowed by the principles that are optimific, uniquely universally willable, and not reasonably rejectable." (2013, 413)

self-evident, and it is the basic norm *to justify* all other middle-level principles from which we can extract particular rules.[44]

Having stated the FEP, we can now take a step further; that is, we can show how care and respect are in tension, but eventually form a unified whole, which is the bulk of *a* CS-Morality. The first thing to be said, then, is that, on the one hand, the basic idea of most versions of rule-consequentialism is that everyone's well-being matters and matters equally, and, accordingly, we must care for everyone equally even if we need to give *some* priority to those close to us (a rule making this permissible brings the best consequences and justice seems to have nothing against it); on the other hand, the Kantian idea of respect for persons or a rights-based theory cannot be taken in negative terms as possessing negative rights only, but involves considering any person's ends as my own incrementing her positive rights. Consequently, it is everyone's duty to promote any person's well-being.

Now, some philosophers have argued that care ethics or virtue ethics is just a *supplement* to a principled ethics, but, formally considered, virtue ethics can be incorporated into the fundamental principle of morality. That is to say, according to virtue ethics, an act is right if and only if it is the kind of act a virtuous character would perform in the circumstances. My proposed amended Triple Theory incorporates all three *formal* elements of the main normative ethical theories, namely rule-consequentialism, moderate forms of deontology and most versions of virtue ethics, into the fundamental principle of *a* CS-Morality. Therefore, in proposing the integration of care and respect we must be crystal clear as to what is accomplished. The first misunderstanding that must be avoided is that of *reductionism*: the idea is *not* to subsume one notion into the other. More importantly, by desiring to keep these two notions distinct, the main purpose is to show that they are not incompatible and exclusive. Care and respect are in fact complementary moral attitudes as one can recognize in the concept of *caring respect*.

I would then like to discuss now whether the language of care can *mutatis mutandis* be fully translated into that of respect for rights and vice-versa. As some care theorists have argued, we can construct an argument to

[44] As I pointed out in the Introduction, given that we are considering neurobioethics as based on a philosophical search for wisdom, finding a first ethical principle is crucial to such an enterprise. As Aristotle wrote: "wisdom must plainly be the most finished of the forms of knowledge. It follows that the wise man must not only know what follows from the first principles, but must also possess truth about the first principles." (EN 1141^{a}17) I consider this first principle a hinge-proposition in a Wittgensteinian sense. It has a clear justificatory role in neurobio*ethics* overcoming the weakness of the meta-ethical intuitionist assumptions of principlism.

show that persons have an obligation to care and consequently to show that all individuals have a right to be cared for (Engster 2009, 53). We could also argue that we can arrive at most of the requirements of care using the language of rights. As the feminist philosopher Virginia Held puts it (2006, 69): "We could then recognize basic well-being, or welfare, as something to which each person is entitled by right under conditions of need and ability of the society to provide. Welfare rights would be recognized as basic rights guaranteeing persons the resources needed to live." I believe this is true, and we must insist upon this possibility without pretending to reduce care to respect. By the way, it is not clear how Held herself manages to integrate care and justice. Contrary to her own official view, she still seems sometimes to think of care as being more related to the private domain, whereas respect for rights or justice is more related to the public domain. I think that the best way to avoid such misunderstandings is, however, to focus on the object of care (*the well-being* of vulnerable individuals such as the deprived, the very young, the elderly, the sick etc.) and the object of respect (*the personhood* of autonomous agents, who need to care for themselves). In this way, we can overcome the polarizations of private/public and male/female. It seems mistaken then to reduce either respect to caring or vice versa. It is better to keep these notions distinct, so we can see when *they limit each other*, preventing paternalism and indifference.

It becomes easy to see that care and respect are two sides of the same coin: the bulk of *a* CS-Morality. As I argued above, much of the language of care could be translated into the language of rights (e.g., caring not to harm into a right not to be harmed). But not all contents of care are exhausted by a system of intrinsic rights. An individual's well-being has many contingent factors and even the best rights system cannot anticipate all the necessities a person will have throughout her life. This is another reason to keep both concepts, care and respect, as the basic cornerstones of *a* CS-Morality in the search for a unified approach.

In order to achieve this unified view, it is crucial then to bear in mind that respect is *not* a purely negative attitude, which commands persons to keep themselves *at a distance* from one another.[45] Thus, a universal ethics of respect cannot be a minimal one. If this were the case, then we would have indifference and a minimal morality based on negative rights only, that

[45] To quote Kant on this point (6: 449): "The principle of **mutual love** admonishes them [human beings] constantly to *come closer* to one another; that of the **respect** they owe one another, to keep themselves *at a distance* from one another." It does not follow, however, that they cannot be integrated showing that views such as Engelhardt's autonomism are mistaken.

is, of non-interference such as not to be harmed, not to be unfairly arrested, etc. But even in a morality based on universal respect, we can find a positive characterization of this moral attitude. To use again Kant's own way of expressing it:

> Humanity might indeed subsist if no one contributed to the happiness of others but yet did not intentionally withdraw anything from it; but there is still only a negative and not a positive agreement with *humanity as an end in itself* unless everyone also tries, as far as he can, to further the ends of others. For, the ends of a subject who is an end in itself must as far as possible be also *my* ends, if that representation is to have its *full* effect in me. (GMM 4: 431)

That is to say, even Kant, who thought that happiness could not be the foundation of morality, held that we have a duty to improve, as our own end, other persons' well-being *for their own sake*.

I have already presented the necessary and hopefully sufficient conditions for the concept of respectful care in the canonical way. Recalling Nodding's attempt, the challenge is now distinct but interconnected. Thus, bearing in mind the previous examination of "care" and "respect," I would like to ask under which conditions a person W (a researcher) *knows-how* to respect Y (e.g., Aysha) in a caring way. This seems to be the case iff:

(i) W recognizes Y as a person, but also sympathizes with her;
(ii) Y has, among others, a basic right to be assisted (e.g., in a fair healthcare system);
(iii) W has learned to fulfill her obligations benefiting Y's for *her* own sake.

Once these conditions are met, respect manifests itself in a caring manner. This is not a *negative* attitude only as proposed by autonomists. The general conclusion, then, is that respect without care is empty; that is, it leads to indifference, which may be the cause of malpractice such as negligence. Since caring respect is the other face of the same coin, it helps to avoid the problems of care without respect, especially paternalistic actions, which are also the cause of much malpractice in neurobioethics. Appealing, now, to the first principle of ethics, we may show that caring respect is optimific, universally willable and would not be rejected by a virtuous person, and is, therefore, plainly justified as a moral attitude.

To illustrate how to apply caring respect, I would then like to go back to our case.[46] Thus, this seems the best place to try briefly to answer two more of the questions formulated by the O3 group mentioned in the Introduction, namely: how should a decision to deploy medical interventions which directly affect the human mind be made? (question 2) Such interventions raise questions about what role, if any, they should have in the criminal justice system, and whether their use would unacceptably threaten human freedom (question 3). Now, regarding the first issue and recalling the Aysha case, I see no need to change the way medical decisions are made as long as they follow basic norms leading to *caring respect*. That means decisions must be made together with the patient (or her representatives). As we have pointed out elsewhere (Dall'Agnol & de Azevedo, 2019), shared decisions lead to the best possible outcome. If a consensus is not reached, one could then appeal to other institutional arrangements, for example, IRBs (Institutional Review Boards) or ethics committees, but we need also to apply caring respect and redefine the main roles of such mechanisms.[47]As it is wellknown, there is a discussion about whether they should have an *advisory* function only or a *decisionary* role too. It seems, however, that their main functions include: to review difficult cases to confirm or not the diagnosis/prognosis; to provide a forum for discussing ethical issues; to formulate policies and guidelines; etc. But, if the concept presented above is sound, then their main role is to ensure that *caring respect* is always in place. It emphasizes the educational role of teaching professional staff *to know-how* to care respectfully or *to know-how* to respect in a caring manner: intrinsically valuing the cared for.

The role of the criminal justice system may basically remain the same as long as it is based on the rule of law. By the "rule of law" I mean the middle level principle, which prescribes that all persons must be

---

[46] The remarks that follow are just preliminary *illustrations* of how we can apply the new moral epistemology developed in the first chapter to guide normative ethics, based on care and respect (integrated into the concept of caring respect) to practical neurobioethical issues. The next chapter will focus on applied ethics and give more examples.

[47] Under the title "Ethical Neuroscience," *Nature Neuroscience* published (Feb. 2010) there is an interesting Editorial calling attention to the need for more coordination and a more transparent decision-making process. The point is "…that ethical review is indeed doing what it sets out to do, by ensuring the welfare of subjects while advancing our knowledge or how the human brain works." Its concern is growing given that in research carried out by private companies, the ethical standards for human subjects do not always follow clear ethical guidelines (e.g., Nuremberg Code; the Helsinki Declaration; the *Belmont Report* [US]; the Res. 466/12 [BR], etc.)

governed by a fair system of public rules specifying rights and obligations and establishing the elements of the common good, enacted by a competent legislative authority, democratically voted for by all citizens and applied in litigation cases by impartial judges in fair trials. If that is in place, we do not need to change the role of the criminal justice system in dealing with neurobioethical challenges.[48] No doubt, human freedom must be protected by the law and neurotechnology cannot be used to violate this and enslave persons.

Paternalism is not only a moral problem; it is a *political* one too. Thus, to finish this section, I would like to remove a political obstacle to thinking and living in terms of a respectful caring or a caring respect attitude, both particularly in neurobioethics and, more generally, in all domains of life. As some political philosophers have pointed out, what gives legitimacy to a government is "equal concern and respect."[49] Dworkin's political principle could be rephrased in terms of "respectful care and caring respect" and be used to analyze the political implications of the concept I have constructed in this section. As I pointed out above, by developing concepts such as caring respect, we arrive at a way of establishing a middle level principle that provides reasons to institute a state and to justify government. This principle can be put in Dworkinian terms: *a government has legitimacy if it treats everyone with the same care and respect*. This principle provides a moral justification for politics, that is, for the institution of a state and a special form of government, namely agonistic democracy. I will return to this point in the next chapter, discussing the institutionalization of neurobioethics in the last section.

Finally, I would now like to synthetize the main achievements of this chapter regarding the idea of *a* CS-Morality. As we have seen, such a system is based on a formal first principle and on the contends of both care and respect. *A* CS-morality is shara*ble* because not all existing value systems may contain the elements of a public moral system and must therefore incorporate them into their own practices. Thus, it is easy to think

---

[48] On this issue, see the Green's and Cohen work "For the Law, Neuroscience Changes Nothing and Everything." (cf. Illes, J. & Sahakian, B., 2013, 655) Of course, there are implications from neuroethics to the law, especially using biomarkers to identify potential mental disorders, that is, it may enhance or reduce legal responsibility. On this point, see: Baum, M. L. *The Neuroethics of Biomarkers*. (Oxford: Oxford University Press), pp. 91-142.

[49] Since his first works, Ronald Dworkin (1977, pp.180-183; 223-39) has argued that there is a basic right to "equal concern and respect" owed to human beings as moral persons. It justifies government and public policies such as the ones I will sort out in the next chapter.

of a caring culture which does not respect the right to self-determination leading to paternalism. That is why it would need to incorporate the main tenets of *a* CS-Morality. This system is not an absolute morality, *the* true, immutable and eternal morality, but a necessary one to prevent pluralism turning into anything-goes-relativism. It has therefore a sound rationale: if we really want to co-exist pacifically, one of the main political aims of living in society, and if we want to flourish through many forms of cooperation (industry, commerce, sports, etc.), and if we want to lead our own personal lives based on our own beliefs, customs, etc., constitutive of our worldview, which is one among many, then there is no option but to subscribe to a *public* morality. I have called this system "*a* CS- morality," ethically supported by a FEP.[50] Consequently, if we want to prevent pluralism turning into normative relativism, having as a consequence the prospect of permanent conflict or even a war of all against all, bringing only devastation, violent outcomes, increased fear, etc., we must endorse such a moral system. *A* CS-Morality is the best way of integrating care and respect in terms of respectful care or, what turns out to be the same, a caring respect attitude.

In the next chapter, I will apply the concept of caring respect to particular (neuro)bioethical issues.

---

[50] Recalling also the results of the previous chapter, we can say that a person *knows-how* to act rightly when she follows norms justified by the first ethical principle. Here, the new moral epistemology of practical cognitivism and the normative ethics of *a* CS-Morality fit well.

CHAPTER 3

APPLIED ETHICS: CARING RESPECT IN NEUROBIOETHICS

We have so far reached two main results in this work: one is meta-ethical and the other normative. The meta-ethical outcome achieved in chapter 1 was the proposal of practical cognitivism as a new moral epistemology capable of overcoming the main problems of the intuitionist basis of the predominant normative approach in bioethics and, arguably, in neuroethics, leading to neurobioethics. Based on the conception of philosophy as a search for wisdom, I argued that moral knowledge is a *sui generis* cognitive phenomenon not reducible to factual or empirical investigations. Thus, a practical cognitivist holds that acting morally involves to *know-how* ϕing, for instance, respecting a person in a certain way, namely in a caring manner. When we substitute the meta-ethics of the *Belmont Report* for practical cognitivism, we may avoid its inherent difficulties, especially the conflicts between middle level norms, which lead to irresolvable moral dilemmas affecting also the predominant bioethical theory: principlism. Practical cognitivism allows us also to see that the concept of "*neuro*ethics" may, when seen only from the perspective of a science of morality, involve a category mistake by misrepresenting descriptive knowledge as prescriptive.

The normative result worked out in chapter 2 was, based on the failure of neuroscience to provide us with a normative framework, to propose *a* CS-Morality based on two fundamental ways of intrinsically valuing, namely, caring for vulnerable beings and respecting persons. These two notions, despite their apparent tensions, may lead to moral attitudes such as caring respect justified by the FEP. In the last section, then, I sorted out the necessary (and hopefully) sufficient conditions to attribute such a moral attitude. Thus, a morality based on respect does not lead to indifference or individualism. This result fits well with the Belmont normative framework which requires us to respect *persons* in doing scientific research using human subjects. This conceptual analysis of caring respect is one of the main normative contributions of this work. It allowed us to reshape the field of neuro*ethics*, understood as the ethics of doing neuroscientific research and neurotechnological experiments, in the direction of neurobioethics and answer some of the questions raised in the introduction of this work.

I would, in this final chapter, like to explore in a more detailed way some of the practical implications of the concept of *caring respect* for neurobioethics to illustrate how it might work in practice. To achieve this aim, I will use the main moral concerns posed by neuroscience and ask whether it really brings new ethical challenges. Afterwards, I will, only in order to illustrate the meta-ethical and normative results of the two previous chapters, focus on the issue of the moral permissibility of using cognitive enhancers and other moral issues related to caring for and respecting a person such as Aysha. To avoid generalizations, I will focus on whether cognitive enhancers are morally permissible and some related neurobioethical issues, for instance, associated mental disorders.

3.1 – New ethical challenges from neuroscience?

What are the real new ethical challenges (if any) the development of the neurosciences and associated neurotechnologies have brought us? To recognize some of the ethical issues, I would like to make more explicit the main topics addressed by the *Global Consortium O3*. The main ethical tasks of the O3 group can be sorted into three main categories: First, there is the challenge of neurotechnology; that is, advances in the biological and neurosciences show great potential for not only treating neurological and psychiatric conditions, but also the possibility of *reading human minds*. Consider, for instance, the use of fMRI for disorders of consciousness. Now, consciousness is often understood to be a marker of personhood, and it is central to an individual's quality of life. Accordingly, end-of-life medical decisions take assessments of consciousness into account (e.g., on the permissibility of euthanasia). However, while significant obstacles still remain, brain-decoding technology could be used to develop devices capable of reading other people's thoughts. Such devices would be of interest to law enforcement agencies, but they could significantly invade an individual's privacy and mental integrity. Here there is an ethical issue that might gain clarity from a neurobioethics based on a caring respectful attitude. The same reasoning applies *to brain-computer interfaces* (BCIs) since they go beyond the observation of brain activity to allow such activity to be translated into commands for computers, and ultimately to control devices of various sorts. Such technology is already of therapeutic interest as BCI advances will allow for the development of neuroprosthetic limbs. As well as raising main neurobioethical issues, BCIs also present novel legal contests: neuroprosthetics challenges the traditional legal dichotomy between body and property; direct mind control of devices tests the distinction between the mental elements and physical elements of a crime, as intention and action merge. Moreover, the possibility of *predicting behavior* brings another domain of questions: neuroimaging is increasingly being investigated as a predictive tool for specific human behaviors, particularly criminal ones. Recent fMRI studies have shown that prisoners who have low activity in the anterior cingulate cortex are more likely to re-offend. Neuroimaging might plausibly come to have far more predictive power than our currently employed risk assessment tools. The crucial question is whether the normative framework presented in the last chapter is capable of dealing with these practical issues. There is no apparent reason why not.

Second, we must consider the potential for controlling and modifying human experience and behavior. Brain stimulation techniques, that is, electrical and magnetic methods of neurostimulation, such as transcranial direct current stimulation (tDCS), transcranial magnetic stimulation (TMS) and deep brain stimulation (DBS) have been used as therapeutic interventions in the treatment of neurological and psychiatric disorders. Some forms of neurostimulation are commercially available, and some, such as tDCS, may even be built by following instructions available on the internet. In the future, optogenetics offers the prospect of increasingly fine grained and profound brain modulation that might furnish us with the ability to exert greater, and more precise, degrees of control over which desires move us, or others, to act. As well as raising ethical questions about the effects of neurostimulation on human agency and personal identity, the possibility of "DIY neurostimulation (tDCS)" raises regulative issues. The use of *cognitive enhancers* already prompts lots of ethical questions since drugs such as amphetamine, methylphenidate, modafinil, etc. (which I will analyse in the next section) are apparently improving human performance. Consider also *mood and emotional alteration*: psychedelic states have long been a part of religious and cultural traditions. There is an ever-increasing number of drugs which could modify mood and conscious states. Moreover, oxytocin may, with some limitations, increase the human ability to foster altruistic relationships.[51] Does the fact that these altered states and enhanced

---

[51] We must, however, be cautious on this point. Many studies (De Dreu 2011, 1262f.; Greene 2013, 54; Cortina 2018, 223) call attention to the fact that oxytocin, a neurotransmitter and hormone that is involved in maternal care and was previously believed to increase empathy and trust only, is also associated with in-group favoritism and even sectarism. This is a good example of how a quick transposition

relationships have been facilitated by neuro-interventions undermine the contribution that they can make to genuine human well-being? Or take the issue of *moral enhancement*: the fruits of neuroscience have been used to modify human moral behavior. For example, cognitive behavioral therapy, neurofeedback drugs have frequently been used in the treatment of impulsive aggression. More controversially, serious sexual offenders in some jurisdictions are mandated to take anti-libidinal agents in order to reduce their risk or re-offending. Research suggests that other pharmacological agents and neurostimulation could also be used to affect traits that are linked to criminal behavior. Now, for reasons of space, I will focus primarily on the issue of cognitive enhancement in the next two sections to illustrate what the concept of caring respect requires in actual practice and in some institutional arrangements.

Third, there are ethical issues surrounding automated systems for mental health and well-being. Consider, for instance, the use of apps: there has recently been a proliferation of apps designed to treat or to improve mental health and well-being. The goal of these apps is to achieve fully automated "therapies" in which machine-learning algorithms "treat" the patient. Although this would increase access to mental health care, existing apps are unregulated and largely untested, though highly accessible. Consider virtual reality: the advent of affordable mobile virtual reality (VR) headsets has raised the prospect of the use of this technology in mental health care and well-being. VR could allow for decentralized treatment, again increasing access to mental health care. However, there is currently a lack of clinical evidence to support either the routine clinical use of VR, or its use as a "telemedicine." Most promising are care-bots, that is, automated systems that could be developed to provide care and companionship to socially isolated patients, such as the elderly. An interesting question here is whether we can program a respectful caring or a caring respectful robot.

To deal with all these issues goes, undoubtedly, beyond the limits of this work. The O3 itself is a 5-year research group for (2018-2021), with the possibility of an extension of 5 years more.[52] Besides, there are many other issues for a proper philosophy of neuroscience, including questions associated with "neuroethics" such aswhether there is free will or whether neurodeterminism is true (following Lybet's famous experiments); whether

---

from the neuroscience of morality to ethics may lead to a categorial mistake considering oxytocin "the moral molecule" (Zak, 2012).

[52] On the same spirit, it is worth recalling that the B.R.A.I.N. Initiative is planning to spend billions of dollars to map the human brain by 2025. Many scientific discoveries and tecnological applications will certainly emerge, as well as ethical challenges.

the mind is *reducible* to the brain (dualism *vs*. monism); whether –to put in the words of Swaab's and Gabriel's book titles–"we are our brains" or "I am not a brain," that is, issues surrounding personal identity; questions on the relationship between reason and emotions in moral deliberation and decision-making processes as they occur in our nervous system or in society at large, etc. As a philosopher, I believe that, in order to deal properly with all these issues, we must have a sound philosophy of neuroscience, but presenting its main tenets in detail is not my aim in this book.

I would, however, like to mention briefly once again the co-work done by the neuroscientist M.R. Bennett and the philosopher P.M.S. Hacker. I am most sympathetic with their distinction between the empirical investigations of neuroscience and the conceptual work that needs to be done by philosophers.[53] It was in this spirit that I presented a conceptual analysis of "caring respect" in the last chapter in which I referred to a fundamental moral attitude in neurobioethics. Moreover, I do agree with their criticism of the mainstream reductionist approach in neuroscience as represented, for instance, by Patricia Churchland's work in neurophilosophy, which is based on metaphysical naturalism, or Francis Crick's astonishing hypothesis.[54] Basically, I think that eliminative reductionism as presupposed by some neuroscientists leads to scientificism, which is as metaphysical a view. Thus, Bennet and Hacker are right in pointing out, in a very Wittgensteinian spirit, that there is no such thing as "explaining the world," that science is not the measure of all things, and that there are forms of explanation and understanding that are neither scientific nor theoretical. Thus, neuroreductionisms end up, to use Bennett and Hacker's expression (2003, 372), "eliminating all that is human." A scientist's approach to the person ends up removing, for instance, *personhood,* with it being considered even an illusion (Farah 2010, 321), and therefore having supposedly no need to respect a persons' rights.

---

[53] For a critical discussion on Bennett and Hacker's views, see the excellent book *Neuroscience and Philosophy: Brain, Mind, and Language*, organized as a debate between Maxwell Bennett, Daniel Dennett, Peter Hacker and John Searle (cf. References). After all, despite not agreeing with everything they argued for (I still think that knowing-that and knowing-how are two *kinds* of knowledge), I stand by Bennett and Hacker's main philosophical theses.

[54] The astonishing hypothesis, according to Crick (1995, 3), is that "'You', your joys and your sorrows, your memories and your ambitions, your sense of personal identity and free will, are in fact no more than the behavior of a vast assembly of nerve cells and their associated molecules." This is scientificism in its crudest form. It excludes from an individual's biography all personal and social experiences, which are unique to each of us as persons.

As a philosopher, then, I would like to insist upon the *protagonist* role of wisdom, ethically shaped, as a guide for our actions. This means that we should embrace *agnosticism* (not scientificism or any other fundamentalism) when dealing with metaphysical issues, leading to pluralism, which does not mean extreme relativism (*antagonism*) or even radical skepticism. Thus, as I argued in the first chapter, practical *cognitivism* in ethics helps to build up *a* CS-Morality based on mutual care and reciprocal respect capable of justifying the rule of law for a democratic political system as well as being applied in neurobioethical practical issues, as we will see presently in my discussion of cognitive enhancement. This means that in doing neuroscience one can (and certainly must) embrace a *methodological* naturalist approach, but not the reductionist *metaphysical* one expressed in Swaab'sfamous book: *We Are Our Brains*. In other words, we need to avoid "neurocentrism". After the decade of the brain in the 1990's and now the B.R.A.I.N Initiative etc., we should regard, to use Bennet and Hacker's words once again, the "human being as a whole." This implies, for instance, an integration of emotions and reason; regarding free will not just as what is going in your brain, but its legal and social conditions, etc. Thus, my own view of the relations between mind and brain is that even if the former is *supervenient* to the latter, as it clearly appears to be, to reduce the mind to the nervous system is to commit a category mistake, which is the basis for a mereological fallacy. That is to say, complex mental states cannot be identified, in terms of biunivocal correlations, with neural states. The mind and the brain are not isomorphic.

The mind needs to be understood in its own terms. That is to say, it cannot be equated with what is going on in our brain only. A sound argument in this direction was recently put forward by the philosopher Markus Gabriel in his work *I Am Not a Brain.*[55]The main thesis of Gabriel's book is

> … the claim that the human mind engenders an open multiplicity of capacities all of which involve the mind, because the mind creates an image of itself by way of these self-interpretations. *The human mind makes an image of itself and thereby engenders a multiplicity of mental realities.* This process has a structure that is historically open, and which cannot be conceived only in the language of neurobiology. (Gabriel 2017, 28; italics in the original)

---

[55] Actually, Gabriel's original title in German is *Ich ist nicht Gehirn,* which could be translated into English, despite disrespecting grammar, as *I* is *not a brain*, to give the idea that the mind cannot be identified with the brain.

In other words, Gabriel provides a defense of human freedom against the belief that the brain deprives us of our free will. The mind is *spontaneous* in the sense that it is capable of creating self-conceptions of itself at will. Therefore, the mind is autonomous in relation to the brain.

Gabriel's antinaturalistic approach (I would prefer to use the term "non-naturalist" instead of *anti*naturalist) within the philosophy of mind resembles Bennett and Hacker's critique of neuroscientific reductionism. According to the author of *I Am Not a Brain*, it is not true that everything which exists can be investigated by the natural sciences, so there are immaterial realities. His example is the concept of friendship: when I consider a friend, I do not suppose that the friendship between us is a material thing. I believe that Gabriel is right in arguing against neurocentrism and neuromania, especially against the reductivistic approach. Not only friendship, but many other cultural artefacts, especially moral values such as caring and respecting, cannot be understood by observing what is going on in the brain only. This was Farah's main wrong assumption. There are certainly neural counterpoints to the concept of respectful care or caring respect, but there is no need to check them using fMRI to see what is going on in our brains when we judge whether a particular practice in the healthcare system or a special neuroscientific investigation is following the ethical requirements or not. Does it matter, from a moral point of view, whether it activates part of the limbic system (e.g., the amygdala) or the front of the brain (the cortex) only? I think that, from an ethical point of view, it is irrelevant. That is why *neuro*ethics does not lead to anything normatively relevant; only neurobio*ethics* does. What does matter, therefore, is whether the concept of caring respect is sound enough to hold neuroscientists accountable.

Another way of seeing that the mind is not reducible to the brain is to understand correctly what is sometimes referred to as the *extended mind* hypothesis.[56] I will here adapt this idea to show that the mind is not reducible to the brain. Leaving aside the functionalist parity principle, namely that if the same kind of goals and behaviors are subserved by external processes and mechanisms as they are by internal, they ought to be regarded as the same kind of thing, which may lead us to attribute mental states to, for instance, apps, there is a grain of truth in the externalist view regarding mental states such as beliefs, desires etc. By a "a grain of truth,"

[56] Clark, A. & Chalmers, D. The Extended Mind. *Analysis*. (58), 1998. pp.7-19. See also Menary (2010) for more on the extended mind hypothesis. For a critical discussion on this hypothesis and its neuroethical implications see: Levy, P. Neuroethics and the Extended Mind. In: Illes, J. & Sahakian, B. *The Oxford Handbook of Neuroethics* (Oxford: Oxford University Press, 2013). pp. 285-294.

I mean the fact that there are similarities between, for instance, the human memory of a particular landscape and a photograph of the same landscape stored in a computer, but there are also relevant differences (e.g., in the human mind it may evoke particular feelings). Thus, the functionalistic interpretation of the extended mind is problematic. The internalist view, however, is in no better position. That is to say, it seems clear that the mind *materializes* in many cultural artefacts, including moral values, which are transmitted and transformed from generation to generation. What seems missing also is the free capacity of the mind to create and develop its own pluralistic visions of the world, which are assimilated by "new brains" in all sorts of new ways.To give an ethical example, a social Darwinist may well believe that morality is synonymous with altruistic cooperation only, but a Christian could maintain that morality is a divine commandment for humans, and both will try to inculcate new generations with their worldviews. What is now needed is *a* CS-Morality to make it possible for them to co-exist pacifically, to cooperate, and to respect each other. For that goal, we may use *arguments*, *concepts,* etc., which are not reducible to the biochemistry of the brain, but may have external scaffoldings (this book, for instance). Once again, the mind is not identifiable with the brain, but has spontaneous activities of its own that generates science, culture, religion, arts, and philosophy, and spreads them throughout the social world. We are part of nature, but nurture plays a role in shaping our mental identities *and* our brains.

When I argued that the mind is *supervenient* to the brain, but not reducible to it, one thing that I was implying was that, being free and spontaneous, the mind is capable of generating new *symbolic* art, of *transcending* particular experiences and giving them religious significance, of *imagining* contrafactual hypothesis to produce scientific knowledge, etc., which does not, strictly speaking, belong to the physical world, but is part of our cultural, historical and intersubjective heritage. In other words, the mind is *free* to *create* intersubjective culture, new languages, and so on. Imagination has certainly neural correlates, but its product, for instance an *idea*, has a life of its own. Consequently, it cannot be located in this or that particular brain only. Consider, for instance, the concept of caring respect proposed here: it cannot be identified with the neural correlate events of a particular brain, but has a *normative* significance in guiding our intersubjective actions, which is not reducible to factuality. The same applies to concepts such as rights, responsibilities, persons, etc.; they are not just natural entities like physical objects, but moral and legal notions.

Not everything is, however, lost for neuroscientific applications in ethics. I do agree that the use of neurotechnology can help with neurobioethical issues. Now, in a subsequent work, namely "Personhood, Consciousness, and Severe Brain Damage," Martha J. Farah (2013, 185), this time writing alone, points out that "...functional brain imaging has been used in a variety of ways to better assess *the personhood* of severely brain-damaged patients." (my emphasis) Thus, it appears that she came to recognize that the concept of personhood is not just an illusion after all and in fact plays an important role in ethics. Of course, the concept is difficult to define and many criteria could be considered: rationality, agency, self-awareness, cognition about the future, linguistic communication, consciousness, etc. But the difficulties in defining personhood are not sufficient to declare it a fantasy. Many concepts (if not all) are hard to define (e.g., love, justice, etc.), but the issue is rather metatheoretical, that is, what to expect from a definition. Basically, it is a stipulative device for theoretical purposes; it is neither an expedient to state what something really is (real definition) nor an arbitrary one (nominal definition). Thus, what was strange in Farah's and Heberlein's previous work was that, because personhood does not correspond to a category of physical objects in the world, it is just an illusion. Is justice or any other ethical concept an illusion because it does not have the ontological status of a physical object such as a plant? I hope to have presented in this last chapter a cogent argument to refute the thesis that personhood is an illusion making room for rights and the principle of respect for persons.

I am now in a position to state in a clearer way one of the main proposals of this book: if neuroethics, in its ambiguous use, implies a *nihilistic* program based on a positivist conception of neuroscience in getting rid of a morality based on persons, then we need to redirect it entirely to what I have been calling "neurobio*ethics*." That is to say, since most of the so-called neuroethical problems seem to be bioethical ones after all, the Belmont framework must be fully applied to neuroscientists: this is what neurobio*ethics* is mainly about. Consequently, I am *from now on* attaching a specific *ethical* framework to the characterization of neurobioethics. That is to say, my use of "neurobioethics" has a normative side to it, namely I subsume neuroethical issues to neurobio*ethics* to make full sense to this book's title. The plausibility of such redefinition is based not only on the idea that the neuroscience of morality is just *a science* among other empirical sciences of human moral conduct *insufficient* to understand morality as a whole, but mainly that, by using human beings who happen to be persons as subjects of scientific investigation, neuroscientists must answer to the Belmont ethical framework, mainly to the *prima facie* principles of respect for persons (including a right to fair distribution) and beneficence (including non-maleficence) as justified by the *first principle of ethics,* leading to fundamental obligations such as caring respect.

Recalling, then, some of the main concerns of the *Global Consortium O3*, namely the challenges of new neurotechnologies (human mind-reading machines *versus* mental privacy; the potential for controlling and modifying human experience and behavior through smart drugs known as cognitive enhancers (amphetamine, modafinil, etc); the (mis)use of apps for mental health and well-being etc., it seems clear that *neurobioethics* is well equipped to avoid abusive practices. By relying on caring respect (and respectful care) we are better off than if we measure our neuroscientific and neurotecnological achievements using a utilitarian rationality only. As we saw in the previous chapter, recent "neuroscientific" attempts to establish ulitarianism as the normative ethics are not well grounded. Actually, only the FEP of the Triple Theory is capable of justifying fundamental moral attitudes such as caring respect. Now, as we will see in the next section on cognitive enhancers, there is a clear need for more caring and respectful practices.

This result fully supports *Nature Neuroscience's* editorial entitled "The Ethical Neuroscientist."[57]According to the editors, there is a growing concern regarding the violation of regulations. For instance, in the drug-testing business, it is reported that companies are using immigrants to participate in trials and that subjects are not given adequate care. I will discuss this point in relation to cognitive enhancers as an illustration of the need for more caring respect, but it is against the Belmont's recommendations to select "undesirable" persons for risky research. It is clearly an uncaring and disrespectful attitude; the very opposite to what is required by caring respect in *neurobioethics*.

Finally, it is worth pointing out that I do not pretend to solve all the philosophical issues surrounding neuroscience here, but rather limit myself to the ethics of performing such a scientific enterprise and some of its neurotechnological applications. There are many relevant issues I could use to prove that neurobio*ethics*, as above defined, is better than the use of simply "*neuro*ethics." One area of O3's concerns, which I would like to say

---

[57] The editorial explicitly calls for neuroscientists working in the private sector, where they are not required to follow the *Belmont Report* as academics are, to avoid ethical lapses: "Many neuroscientists do both academic and commercial research, and there is no justification for applying different ethical standards, particularly for subject selection and informed consent, in the two areas. To avoid the need for such regulation, we urge all neuroscience research companies to commit to following the *Belmont Report* guidelines and to publicly disclose how they evaluate ethical concerns." *Nature Neuroscience* (March 2008).

something, is the experimental use of drugs for the treatment of mental disorders such as anxiety, depression, dementia, schizophrenia, etc. or for purposes of enhancement, which could be Aysha case. It is time for a well-based criticism of some psychiatric (ab)uses, which lead to the medicalization of life if not to social crises such as the opioid epidemic. In order to avoid generalizations, I would like to focus on the ethical issues related to doing neuroscientific investigations and testing new neurotechnologies that aim at cognitive enhancement.

3.2 – Treatment *versus* cognitive enhancement

In this section, I would like to examine issues surrounding the polemic of treatment *vs*. enhancement, especially cognitive improvement, as a way of testing the moral epistemology and the normative concepts that I worked out in the first two chapters. In order to do that, it is crucial to recall the basic *facts* of the Aysha case presented in the first chapter.

The main *ethical* questions we were asked to investigate are:

(i) Should cognitive enhancers be available to poor people in poor countries?
(ii) Who should pay?
(iii) Is it important to establish the evidence for cognitive enhancement safety and efficacy prior to launching such a programme?
(iv) Who should pay for developing that evidence?
(v) Could widespread, sanctioned cognitive enhancement reinforce stigma and oppression of those who opt in/out?
(vi) Could cognitive enhancement programmes be used to target specific groups for "treatment"?
(vii) Is cognitive capacity just a brain matter; or there are other ways to enhance cognition that should be attended to?

I will throughout this section say a word or two on each of these questions to reconstruct what my view at that time was –and to some extent still is– on these issues, without pretending to present a final answer.

Considering the social and *experimental* nature of such a program, I would like then to test the meta-ethical theory put forward in the first chapter and the normative concept constructed in the second, namely caring respect. First, the idea is to verify whether practical cognitivism is a better meta-ethical foundation for neurobioethics instead of the predominant intuitionist approach. In order to achieve this goal, we must remember that principlism has no clear criterion to avoid dilemmatic situations, and it is, consequently, incapable of guiding our actions effectively. That is why we must *know-how* to apply the first principle of ethics for *a* CS-Morality. We need to correct the meta-ethical problem by using practical cognitivism in the direction of caring and respecting Aysha –and any person indeed– as, so to speak, a whole biopsychosocial unity, even if her prefrontal cortex (reasoning) is not ready to control impulses from the limbic system (especially the amygdala, the center for emotions). I would then like to ask: could we say that such an experimental program, as proposed in the Aysha case, shows real caring respect for the students themselves? To answer this question, I will first use practical cognitivism tied to the first principle of ethics to revise what each middle level norm requires and, second, apply in a more detailed way the concept of caring respect to the case at hand.

To start with, it is necessary to introduce in a clearer way the distinction between treatment and enhancement. Despite the fact that there is a grey area to consider, a sound definition is needed to decide whether public resources must be used for treatment only or for potentializing capabilities as well. No one will doubt that in Aysha's case, if she has cognitive impairments, a new drug should be used as treatment; while for a healthy adult, boosting memory beyond normal functioning using, for instance a nootropic, must be considered enhancement. In other cases, the distinction may not be so clear. Anyway, I would like here to refer to Nick Bostrom and Rebecca Roache's (2011, 138) as well as Anders Sandberg and Julian Savulescu's work (2011, 93) in order to stipulate the following two definitions related to the topic we are analyzing:

> *Cognitive treatment* $=_{\text{def}}$ to fix neuro-impairments such as malfunctioning, degeneration, mental disorders, underperformance etc. of the internal/external processing of information, that is, of the cognitive system;
> *Cognitive enhancement* $=_{\text{def}}$ to boost mental capabilities such as attention, memory etc. beyond normal functioning of the cognitive system.

A treatment then presupposes the existence of a malfunction, a disorder, that is, a subperformance of the cognitive system; enhancement is a clear amelioration of the workings of the normal/natural systems, that is, optimizing their capabilities well beyond their uses for typical individuals of our species.

It is crucial to point out that there are *conventional* ways of enhancing our cognitive capabilities (e.g., via training, formal education) and *non-conventional* means, for instance, the pharmacological ones proposed in the school experiment related above. Since my focus here is on non-conventional means of enhancing cognitive capacities, I will not discuss the conventional ones, which may range from listening to Mozart to improving formal training itself, for instance, enhancing memory by making associations or other mental exercises. Moreover, there are culturally acceptable non-conventional means of improving cognition such as the use of caffeine and nicotine. In many competitive areas such as business, high-performance sports, and even in high schools and colleges many people appeal to smart drugs as enhancers. This raises questions of justice, which will be examined soon. I will not discuss non-conventional forms of cognitive enhancement based on *genetic* interventions here. Given the case presented above, I will limit myself to pharmacological means of enhancing cognitive capabilities. There are, however, new techniques, for instance CRISPR, which will make it possible safely to intervene in the human genome, with the potential to change our brain inducing mental traits such as intelligence and personality. Much also is expected from the current experiments on human brain organoids. Given their complexity, I will not examine these possibilities here, but they have clear ethical and social implications.[58]

With a clear distinction between treatment and enhancement at hand, we may start to discuss what some *existing* pharmaceutical cognitive enhancers (PCEs) could or not do to improve cognitive performance in contexts such as the one presented above. To start by examining the case of Aysha, the first thing to be noted is that it is not clear why the students are not performing well. Granted, the class is overcrowded, the teachers are unmotivated and perhaps underpaid, etc., but this seems not to be sufficient to propose using drugs to enhance cognitive capacities. One of the questions posed by O3 is this: could cognitive enhancement programmes be used to target specific groups for "treatment"? This is a crucial question since treatment seems to have priority over enhancement. Let us, then, suppose for argument's sake that Aysha or some of her colleagues had been diagnosed with a condition such as Attention Deficit-Hyperactivity Disorder (ADHD) or any other similar problem.

First of all, it is important to have a clear understanding of this disorder.[59] According to the DMS-5, in order to be diagnosed with attention deficit (AD) six or more of the following symptoms must have been present for at least *six months*, be inconsistent with the child's developmental level,

---

[58] On this point see Nuffield Council on Bioethics' document *Genome Edition: an ethical review*: http://nuffieldbioethics.org/project/genome-editing

[59] A neurobiological animation explaining ADHD can be found here: https://www.youtube.com/watch?v=4r3XWj269_g

and have a negative effect on their social and academic activities:[60] (i) fails to pay close attention to details; (ii) has trouble sustaining attention; (iii) does not seem to listen when spoken to directly; (iv) fails to follow through on instructions and fails to finish schoolwork or chores; (v) has trouble getting organized; (vi) avoids or dislikes doing things that require sustained focus; (vii) loses things frequently; (viii) is easily distracted by other things; (ix) forgets things. Now, to be diagnosed with Hyperactivity Disorder (HD), six or more of these symptoms must also be present for at least six months, be inconsistent with the child's developmental level, and have a negative effect on their social and academic activities: (i) fidgets with hands/feet or squirms in chair; (ii) frequently leaves chair when sitting is expected; (iii) runs or climbs excessively; (iv) has trouble playing or engaging in activities quietly; (v) acts "on the go" and as if "driven by a motor;" (vi) talks excessively ; (vii) blurts out answers before questions are completed; (viii) has trouble waiting or taking turns; (ix) interrupts or intrudes on what others are doing. ADHD is a combination of these two disorders. It is also worth ponting out that ADHD comes in mild, moderate and severe forms.

In the US, around 6 million children were diagnosed with ADHD in 2016.[61] Among children with ADHD, 62% were taking medication (Ages 2-5: 18%; Ages 6-11: 69%; Ages 12-17: 62%). In recent years in Brazil, the consumption of methylphenidate (commercially known as Ritalin®) to treat ADHD has increased by 775% making the country the second largest consumer in the world.[62] It seems that there is something wrong not only with our children, but perhaps with our educational system and our society as a whole. For obvious reasons there are no final numbers, but, according to Ragan, Bard and Singh (2013, 589), 15% of undergraduates were taking smart drugs in American colleges for not treatment, but simply as cognitive enhancers. What is the danger? Apart from addiction, their absence may

---

[60] As it is perhaps well-known, DSM-V classifies ADHD as a mental disorder (See also ICD-10, the International Classification of Diseases, HKD (hyperkinetic disorder)). It has been treated using amphetamine (the basic ingredient of Adderall®) or methylphenidate (the basic ingredient of Ritalin®). I will discuss this and other mental disorders bellow in greater detail since there is a potential link between a diagnosis of ADHD early in life and developing other mental disorders such as anxiety and depression later on. According to Urban and Gae (2014, 3), treatment with methylphenidate actually *induces* anxiety that persists into adulthood.

[61]The American Psychiatric Association states in the Diagnostic and Statistical Manual of Mental Disorders (DSM-5, 2013) that 5% of children have ADHD, but other studies in the US have estimated higher rates in community samples. Cf. https://www.cdc.gov/ncbddd/adhd/data.html<acess: 04/23/2019>

[62] Source: PhD thesis submitted at the State University of Rio de Janeiro in 2014 by psychologist Denise Barros.

lead to anxiety and depression, which requires new treatments, eventually leading to a vicious circle. I will return these other mental disorders in the next section.

Now, the moral issues surrounding any particular prognostic course of action fall not only under classical medical ethics, but most properly belong to traditional bioethics itself given the *experimental* nature of such a scientific program using human subjects as presented in the above case of Aysha. Consequently, it belongs to the domain of what I, in a sense that must be clear by this point, call neurobio*ethics*. Now, it seems clear that, based on notions of both *care* and *respect*, a neurobioethicist would, based on the first principle of ethics, argue that if Aysha and many of her collegues have ADHD, they need *treatment* and this has, consequently, *priority* over enhancement.

Second, I would now like to ask the following question: what are the current pharmaceutical cognitive enhancers (PCEs) available for treatment and what are the prospects for using them or similar drugs in a school setting as enhancers in a particular state as a public program? Without pretending cover all the existing options, I will briefly scrutinize some of the best known and most debated in the literature by reviewing some works published in collections (see: Farah 2010 [5 chapters]; Savulescu *et al.* 2011 [5 chapters]; Chatterjee & Farah, 2013 [5 chapters]; Illes & Sahakian, 2013 [7 chapters]) and some isolated papers. The main aim is to illustrate how they funcion and discuss whether they can deliver the promise of enhancing normal brain functioning. The PCEs to be presented below tend to affect neurotransmitters such as dopamine, norepinephrine, acetylcholine and serotonin. Apart from the already mentioned methylphenidate, the best known are based on amphetamines, for instance those commercially known as Adderall® (a mixture of salts) and modafinil (known as Provigil® in the US and as Stavigile® in Brazil). Generally speaking, amphetamines improve attention and related psychological factors such as subjective energy, wakefulness, and motivation. They have clear medical uses including speech therapy for aphasic patients, narcolepsy etc. and, of course, ADHD. Modafinil also improves alertness and wakefulness and, more controversially, better decision making. Now, methylphenidate intervenes in the brain increasing a person's arousal, energy level, and attentional focus. As I said above, it is also widely used to treat ADHD.[63] Should they be made *permissible* as enhancers in a wider social context such as in public schools?

---

[63] There are other potential pharmaceutical cognitive enhancers (PCEs) under research: cholinesterase inhibitors also improve attention and memory (Chatterjee 2013, p.5); ampakines contribute to acquisition of long term memories (Sanberg *et*

Before attemping to answer this question, I would like to make it crystal clear that UN Convention of Psychotropic Substances (1971), of which the U.S. and Brazil are signatories, states the following Resolution regarding *Research on the Amphetamine Drugs*:

> The Conference, Considering that the amphetamines are particularly liable to abuse and are objects of illicit traffic, Considering that the therapeutic value of these drugs, though acknowledged, is limited, 1. Requests the World Health Assembly to encourage research on less dangerous substances capable of replacing the amphetamine drugs, and to sponsor such research within the limits of the available resources; 2. Recommends that Governments with the necessary facilities should take similar action.[64]

Article 4 further clarifies that if the substance has the capacity to produce a state of dependence and central nervous system stimulation or depression, resulting, for instance, in hallucinations or disturbances in motor function, thinking, behavior, perception or mood, the necessary measures must be taken to prevent abuses. In what follows, then, one must keep in mind that the use of substances such as amphetamines is illegal for non-therapeutic purposes and that the discussion here is *ethical* as opposed to, for instance, based on the existing laws of a particular jurisdiction.[65] Besides, the above case speculates on the possibility of discovering and testing a *new* drug, a supposedly safe and efficient one, which will be discussed below.

What is, then, morally required by a caring *respectful* attitude in Aysha's case considering the use of existing PCEs? That is to say, should we apply the principle of *respect for persons* or just respect for an autonomous decision? Considering Aysha's age, one of the first issues is whether she is really a full agent capable of making the required choice; that is, being 16 years old, whether she is fully capable of making decisions and being held accountable for them. It seems clear that, even if she is not (and neuroscience has important contributions to make here), we must bear in mind that the principle of *respect for persons* requires us also to protect individuals with diminished autonomy. How then can neuroscience help in

---

al. 2013, p.278; Chatterjee 2013, p.5); acetylcholinesterase inhibitor prescribed as a treatment in Alzheimer's disease has also positive effects on memory functioning in healthy individuals (Farah 2010, p.13; Metzinger & Hildt 2013, p. 249). It goes beyond the objectives of this work to provide a full survey on all existing PCEs.

[64] UN, *The International Drug Control Conventions*, 2013, p.76 (see References).

[65] It is worth calling attention to the fact that Aderall® is not authorized by ANVISA in Brazil. A list, in Portuguese, of prohibited substances might be found here: http://bvsms.saude.gov.br/bvs/saudelegis/svs/1998/prt0344_12_05_1998_rep.html

Aysha's case? Well, for one thing, neuroscientific studies of brain development could aid in establishing whether a teenager is capable of making such an important decision as to whether to use drugs to boost her cognitive capacities. In this sense, empirical evidence shows that the prefrontal cortex, the brain's remote-control center, may not be fully developed until the mid-20s.[66] Thus, neuroscience has clearly shown that teenagers do not have a brain capable of controlling their impulses from their limbic system, which is responsible for *emotional* behavior. Consequently, they have less capacity to give informed consent and are more susceptible to coercion or manipulation as well. This is one crucial way neuroscience can shed some light on the moral and legal ages for responsibility despite the fact that it cannot provide a normative system on its own. It is difficult, however, to say something specific on Aysha's particular condition; some teens may be more mature than others, more informed, etc.

One way out of the difficulty is to consider, as Ilina Singh and Keely Kelleher do in their work "The Case for Clinical Management of Neuroenhancement in Young People," whether teenagers would be able *to assent* instead of giving their *informed consent*. This seems clearly to be the case, but even so, according to the authors of the mentioned paper, "…the rights of parents to determine what is in the best interests of the young persons may take precedence…" (Singh & Kelleher 2013, 23). This solution could, however, generate a new difficulty. As it is well known, not all parents make the best decisions for their children. Granted, Aysha's family has the right to decide whether or not to join the program (if her school decides to participate), but that does not guarantee the best outcome for Aysha *herself*. This means that respecting autonomy is not necessarily respecting the patient or the subject of research herself as a person. Self-determination is *one* right a person has, but there are many others, such as body integrity, equal treatment and so on so forth. Here, once again, we see that principlism fails because of its intuitionist assumptions, and we need

---

[66] Cf. Kotulak, R. Teens Driven to Distraction. *Chicago Tribune*. March 24, 2006. There are many other scientific studies on brain development, including in teenagers. See, for instance, Syngh, I. & Kelleher, K. The Case for Clinical Management of Neuroenhancement in Young People. In: Chatterjee, A. & Farah, S. *Neuroethics in Practice. Medicine, Mind, and Society*. (Oxford: Oxford University Press, 2013), pp.16-34. See also: "Development of the Adolescent Brain: Neuroethical Implications for the Understanding of Executive Function and Social Cognition." (Luciana, M. 2013, p.59f.) One important study was recently done by Urban & Gao (2014) on performance enhancement and brain plasticity in the healthy developing brian, which I will comment in detail soon.

practical cognitivism and the normative concepts developed in the first two chapters. Thus, one clear advantage of considering the principle *respect for persons* is that it avoids these problems because young people do have rights, as the *Belmont Report* makes clear, *to protection* given their greater vulnerability.[67] In other words, they have rights to develop fully their autonomy as persons. Now, it seems clear also that some contextual differences must be taken into consideration. For instance, in the US, if Aysha assents or the parents give their informed consent, then the program could perhaps be implemented more easily, but in Brazil, invoking issues surrounding social justice, the public resources may need to be applied elsewhere. I will return to this point.

A serious concern is that PCEs may change not only the way the brain works, but, most fundamentally, affect our sense of what means to be a person. That is to say, they may change deeply our own understanding of what it means to be human as a moral being. There are worries that PCEs have the effect of altering the *sense of individuality* and even *eroding character*. There is no need to stick to a metaphysical view on the essence of human nature to recognize that inauthentity becomes a real threat, but it does not follow that anything goes. If PCEs are to be permitted at all, they must enlarge our sense of humanity as a moral species, that is, our sense of autonomy, value and personhood, not the reverse. Here we see that an empty, negative conception of respect as represented by Engelhardt's autonomist approach, already criticized in the previous chapters, is insufficient to deal with the moral challenges of PCEs since it leads to moral indifference and political individualism. We must keep in mind that care generates reasons for actions that are agent-neutral and that only a caring respectful attitude is really grounded by the first principle of ethics.

Apart from respecting *persons*, which are the other requirements of a *caring* respectful attitude to be considered in order to decide whether Aysha could engage in pharmacological means for enhancing her brain's capabilities? I would now like to apply *the norms of non-maleficence and beneficence* coinjointly since they are also a core assumption of a *caring* respect. What one needs to do here is basically to balance the costs and risks with potential benefits. The norm is formally sound (B>H). Now, both the

---

[67] According to the documentary "Take your Pills" (Netflix, 2018), most children are diagnosed with ADHD when they are only 6 years old. Astonishingly enough, around 11% of American children are nowadays treated for ADHD. This seems to lead to what is referred to as "medicalization of life." In her comments, Martha Farah makes, however, clear that Adderall® has motivational, not a real cognitive enhancement effect. There are better options for some cases, for instance, more physical exercise, meditation, to learn how to focus, etc.

cost-effectiveness (CEA) and cost-benefits (CBA) methods are widely used, but they contain many evaluative assumptions and leave many open questions. For instance, what is a reasonable risk of a harm's occurrence when taking cognitive enhancers? In the neuroenhancement case, there are many specific issues, but the methods remain basically the same. One should consider the risks of engaging in an experimental cognitive enhancement programand balance them with the potential benefits. Aysha and her colleagues are subject to many risks as Singh and Kelleher (2003, 20) made clear in their work on young people: *the development of psychosis or other psychiatric disorders, appetite suppression, insomnia,exacerbation of pre-existing heart conditions, addiction, growth suppression, stigma,the development of an unauthentic self, etc.* Perhaps the most severe is the long-term unknown impact on brain development from the continuing use of stimulants, or any experimental drug indeed.

Since *addiction* is truly a huge harm, I would like to say a few more words on this issue here. It seems clear that the gravity of addiction makes smart drugs that kick-start motivation and concentration for study something prescrible for medical reasons only, that is, for the treatment of conditions such as ADHD. The consequences, however, of continuous use must also be fully considered. The high probability of addiction constrains the cost-benefit analyses and shows that there are sound reasons to be careful in prescribing psychotropic substances, but also that the permissibility of such drugs for enhancement must be deeply analyzed. Considering all the side-effects pointed out by Singh and Kelleher above, it seems clear that *existing* PCEs cannot be used in a program such as the one presented above. *Ex hypothesi* a new PCE must be safe and efficient; that is, it must also be nonaddictive.[68]

All these potential costs and risks of harms need to be contrasted with the expected benefits. As stated above, they seem also to be the following: an increase in the capacity for concentration, alertness, better motivation, an increased sense of agency, better life prospects, etc. But, despite the fact that many drugs developed to treat disorders such as ADHD are used as cognitive enhancers, for instance in colleges by healthy students (specially, amphetamines), it is becoming clear that they do not provide significant cognitive gains. What they really do is to boost the capacity to focus, and consequently, to study. There is no real improvement in intelligence whatsoever. Therefore, they may generate great (and perhaps false) expectations that cannot be completely fulfilled.

---

[68] According to Chatterjee (2013, p.5), however, "newer nonaddictive drugs such as atomoxetine are likely to increase off-label use of such medications."

There seems to be also social gains as potential benefits of a large scale cognitive enhancement program. *If it is safe* and efficient for individuals, society at large may benefit from *developments in the sciences, innovative technologies, new artistic and cultural movements*, etc. That is why a social experiment such as the one proposed above could perhaps be justified; that is, it would not only bring individual gains, but, most importantly, social benefits. Of course, this needs also to be balanced against possible social risks. The danger of massive psychological and chemical dependence on drugs and social abuse is a real threat and, in some cases, already a sad reality.[69]

Among the possible individual and social benefits there is the prospect of increasing a sense of agency itself, and, consequently, this raises issues regarding responsibility and, possibly, could redefine agency and perhaps even personhood. According to Singh and Kelleher (2013, 22), the issue of personal responsibility is a complex one because studies suggest that younger children taking stimulants attribute success to *their own actions*, but attribute failures to *the drug not working properly*. As pointed out above while discussing one's own sense of personhood, there is, then, the issue of authenticity surrounding the debate too. The use of stimulants for neuroenhancement poses new challenges for how to hold persons accountable when they do not attribute their failures to their own deliberations and choices, but to something external. That is to say, enhancing cognitive capacities may have a clear effect on how one views accountability: the sense of agency may increase (hyperagency) or decrease.

I can now start to answer some of the questions raised at the beginning of this chapter. Regarding question (iii), there is no doubt that it is crucial to establish sound evidence for cognitive enhancement's *safety and efficacy* prior to launching such a public program involving schools and other state resources. Given its experimental nature and, more importantly, its wide social scale, the answer must be clear: if there is no sound scientific data showing that the new drug works or if there is a more efficient means to achieve the same goals, the program should not be supported. The tests could be done primarily on non-human animals but should perhaps be checked on voluntary adult humans before any use by teenagers to improve their school performance. Here the traditional bioethical procedure can be used: from the IRB's reports for scientific research and drug testing to the

---

[69] The opioid epidemic in the US is a clear example of this kind of abuse of pharmacological drugs. For a discussion on how addiction works by affecting the neurotransmitter dopamine and its connection with devaluating accountability see the works "Addiction and Responsibility" and "The Neurobiology of Addiction: Implications for Voluntary Control of Behavior" by Steven E. Hyman (cf. References).

official approval by, in the US's case, the FDA, or, in the Brazilian case, ANVISA. More on the institutional arrangements needed to implement neurobioethics will be discussed in the last section.

There is no doubt also that, in relation to question (v), the program must be used primarily to target specific groups for treatment. Here I think practical cognitivism guided by the first principle of ethics is capable of showing that caring respect requires giving *priority* to treatment over enhancement. That is to say, *knowing-how* to take care of Aysha *herself*, if she has ADHD, requires respecting her as having a greater need for treatment.[70] Moreover, appealing to the FEP (which is absent in the predominant bioethical theory), it seems clear that it is optimific, universally willable and would not be rejected by a virtuous person to give priority to treatment over enhancement.

A very sensitive issue is certainly any stigmatization caused by the use of cognitive enhancers, either as treatment or to improve performance. Thus, regarding question (iv), namely "Could widespread, sanctioned cognitive enhancement reinforce stigma and oppression of those who opt in/out?" the answer is clearly positive, but it is less obvious what we can do to prevent or to avoid it. In a very competitive environment such as a High School, either joining the program or opting out could bring personal disillusion to particular individuals, and they could be subject to teasing or even bullying. Another important moral issue is *coercion*. There are two main points here: first, a student could suffer *implicit* coercion to maintain her position; second, she may experience *explicit* coercion in the sense of new demands of better performance. There is no doubt that students are under pressure and even coercion when academic assignments or grades are the only means to assess their capabilities for well-paid jobs. This raises issues of distributive justice since PCEs may contribute to widening existing inequalities. I will return to this point later when discussing some social policies regarding the use of cognitive enhancers.

Before doing that, however, I need to analyze one more moral requirement based on respect and ask whether practical cognitivism and the first principle of ethics would not require us to prioritize *justice* to provide real caring respect. Now, justice is one of the most complex ethical

---

[70] Regarding question (vii), since a practical cognitivist holds that there is not only informational knowledge, it seems clear that cognition is not just a brain matter of processing true or false propositions, but requires a wide range of training to develop the relevant capabilities, that is, *knowing-how* to ϕing. Unfortunately, I cannot develop further this point here, but we must bear in mind that we are dealing with very complex educational issues and that the formation of the person as a whole (and not her cognitive capabilities only) must be the main pedagogical goal.

concepts. It seems clear that cognitive enhancers could, if legalized, bring further advantage to those who can afford to buy them, so the issue of economic inequality always looms around the discussion. But whether one sees this as fair or otherwise depends on an ethico-political theory. Now, formally, the Aristotelian fairness requirement for distributing a good (= =; ≠≠) seems unproblematic. There are, however, many different conceptions of justice that play a role in the bioethical field, and it seems impossible to reach a consensus on a *material* criterion to distribute basic goods: libertarians, egalitarians, socialists, etc. are in deep disagreement on this issue. The problem is what criteria(on) we should use to make a fair discrimination: merit, basic necessities, the laws of the market, etc. Besides, there is also the discussion among prioritarianists, sufficintarists etc.

There is no space, obviously, to critically assess all these alternatives here. I will, then, limit myself to examining a proposal made by Anders Sandberg and Julian Savulescu (2011, 103-106) in their article "The Social and Economic Impacts of Cognitive Enhancement" regarding the fairness of using cognitive enhancers. In a subsection "Injustice", the authors, after recognizing that perhaps one of the best objections to enhancers is that they violate the fair criteria of distributive justice (e.g., using public resources to increase a minority's abilities instead of the majority's well-being), speculate which normative theory of justice is best suited to debating the permissibility of cognitive enhancers. They conclude that libertarians would not see anything unfair in developing new drugs with private funds to be distributed by the market, even if the gap between rich and poor increased, while others would argue that the less privileged must have priority to avoid increased inequalities. Since it is unlikely that a theoretical consensus will be reached any time soon, Sandberg and Savulescu switch their focus to the debate on a reasonable starting-point, namely that everyone has a *right to a fair go*, which, so they believe, is independent of political differences regarding theories of justice. To illustrate, they give the following example: supposing that an IQ of 100 is necessary for a great number of social opportunities, including access to higher education or most well-paid jobs, then it would be morally permissible to use cognitive enhancers for persons below that threshold (around 50% of the population) to give them a fair competitive start. Consequently, non-conventional ways of cognitively enhancing a person's capabilities would not be seen as unfair.[71] Besides, according to Sandberg

[71] As Partridge, Lucke and Hall pointed out (2012), however, there is evidence that public opinion does not support legalizing doping in sports and non-conventional ways of enhancing cognitive capabilies. PCE's are, as doping is, considered cheating. See also Doghe *et al* (2012). I owe references on this point to an

and Savulescu, this way of seeing the issue would help us to realize that cognitive enhancers can actually *promote* justice. Consequently, if cognitive enhancers are well administered, they could aid in diminishing injustices and alleviating social and economic inequalities.

Invoking now practical cognitivism and the concept of *caring respect*, as they were developed in the preceding chapters, what can we say on this issue? First, I believe that Sandberg and Savulescu's view is worth considering despite the fact that I disagree on the supposed neutrality regarding theories of justice. Besides, it is worth keeping in mind that existing PCEs do not boost IQ, but only enhance memory. Now, generally speaking, using equal opportunities as a fair starting point is one of the basic assumptions of the egalitarian theory of justice *a la* Rawls, which would not the shared by a libertarian if it were supported by public education, a social healthcare system, etc. This is, however, not a huge problem since it is possible to show that a libertarian political philosophy makes an unsound anthropological assumption as no human being can take care of himself in all domains of life. Besides, I believe that it is important also to realize that Rawls himself came to recognize that we must give priority to those who do not have their basic needs satisfied *before* discussing liberties and equal opportunities. This point will be explored further in the next section on the institutionalization of neurobioethics.

After applying the notions of care and respect guided by practical cognitivism and the first principle of ethics, we are finally in a position to say something more specific on what a *caring respectful* attitude towards Aysha is all about. Now, given that neuroscience shows that Aysha is not fully autonomous in making a decision, the negative consequences (specially, addiction) override the possible benefits, and given that justice requires prioritizing treatment over enhancement, we may conclude that such a public program should not yet be made available by governments using *existing* or similar PCEs.

There is, however, a stronger reason not to support a largescale cognitive enhancement program in schools. Recent studies have shown that using enhancers in the healthy juvenile brain through low doses of methylphenidate, despite appearing to increase cognition or, at least attention, results in impaired WM (working memory) and behavioral

---

anonymous referee of this book. Besides, we must bear in mind that Martha Farah showed that *existing* PCE's do not really increase IQ, but have a motivational effect only, for instance students will focus more and spend longer periods studying to get better grades.

inflexibility (Urban and Gao 2014, 3).[72] Adolescents' prefrontal cortext (PFC) is not fully developed which means there is a high level of plasticity —possibly a product of the slow maturation of this area. The PFC is the center of judgment and control, behavioral inhibition, working memory, decision making, etc. Anything which affects the neurodevelopment of the PFC means a loss of agency and, consequently, what it means to be a person. Thus, compromising someone's PFC causes such severe damage that this alone is sufficient to be against the program envisaged above. It would affect Aysha's and her colleagues' neurodevelopment as a whole person. Flexibility is needed in several domains of life, and to compromise the brain's PFC plasticity means in the end to affect one's personhood. This does not bring the best consequences, cannot be universalized, and it is certainly not what a virtuous person would do.

This is perhaps the best place then to answer questions (i) and (ii) posed by the O3 group regarding Aysha's case, namely: Should cognitive enhancers be available to poor people in poor countries and who should pay? At first I thought "Why not?," but now I see clearly, given the results of this section, especially where compromising the PFC's plasticity is concerned, that existing PCEs *must not* be used as enhancers by young, healthy students. The main reason is that their effects on the PFC's plasticity affects the students' agency and, consequently, personhood itself.

Before concluding, however, once and for all, that any cognitive enhancer should be permanently prohibited, we should bear in mind that the hypothetical case presented at the beginning of this chapter proposes considering a *new* drug, which is, *ex hypothesis* safe and efficient. To finish this section, then, I would like to take this possibility seriously in a different environment and for a different public. That is to say, let us consider the permissibility of cognitive enhancers for healthly adults only.

Leaving the above state program aside for the moment, I would like to propose the following hypothetical case: *what if* scientists find, after years of painstaking research, a new, natural psychoactive substance in the Amazon forest that boosts cognitive ability without presenting the main negative side effects of existing PCEs? Let us call it "Spiritin." It does not only enhance memory, but it also enormously increases creativity. We do not need to discuss the neurobiological basis of creativity here. It is

---

[72] According to Urban and Gao (2014, 3) "reducing NR2B levels without altering NR2A levels, as was seen following juvenile MPH treatment, was enough to alter the direction of PFC long-term plasticity." That is to say, giving children methylphenidate, modafil etc. who do not have ADHD will make them appear to be paying attention to the teacher, less hyperactive and learning might improve, but will also affect their behavioral flexibility damaging their brain forever.

sufficient to consider Spiritin safe and efficient, and most importantly, nonaddictive. It has been tested on rats and humans and is now under analysis for governmental authorization (FDA or ANVISA) to be commercialized.

I believe that most would say that caring *respect* would not make Spiritin morally impermissible for adults. That is to say, we cannot use practical cognitivism and the first principle of ethics to conclude that Spiritin must not be used by healthy adults using their own private resources to accomplish their life projects. Despite that, it is also worth highlighting that many neurobioethical questions remain open to further investigation, especially the issue surrounding *trade-offs*, that is, between using a drug to enhance one ability (memory) at the cost of decreasing another (creativity) or vice-versa (Urban & Gao 2014, 5). Several issues are currently under investigation: is it only possible to enhance one attribute at the cost of diminishing the other? Is it not possible to boost the brain as a whole? That is why, we must, if such a drug is eventually developed, consider what measures we must take to guarantee *caring* respect for those who take it.

A serious discussion on the permissibility of new, safe and efficient nootropics that enhance particular capabilities at the price of diminishing others (the trade-off issue surrounding cognitive enhancement) needs to take into consideration the many life projects people have and the political arrangements necessary to fulfil them. That is to say, healthy adults may take the risk of losing some ability in order to maximize the performance needed for their lives. For instance, an artist may appreciate Spiritin more than someone who needs long-term memory for her work. This again raises ethical questions around the problem of justice, so I will discuss them below. In any case, new drugs such as Spiritin must always be used under medical supervision. Thus, I would like in the last section to discuss some institutional arrangements for providing *caring* respect (and respectful care) for *a* CS-Morality.

3.3 –Institutionalizing neurobioethics

One of the main justifications neuroethicists such as Martha Farah and Steven Hyman gave to create a new field, separate from bioethics, was that the brain and the mind are so special that we need a new name and that neuroscience gives us unprecedented ways of explaining the former and *controlling* the later. In this work, however, I have argued that *neuro*ethics (understood as the neuroscience of ethics) is in fact unable to deliver a normative ethics capable of dealing adequately with the ethics of neuroscientific studies using human beings as subjects (neuro*ethics*), and that we need to appeal to traditional bioethics to provide normative guidance. Moreover, I have proposed adding neuroethical issues to the subfield of bioethics, and that it would, based on principles such as respect for persons, be sufficient to face the main moral challenges so far in neuroscience and neurotechnology.

In this last section, I would like to examine more closely what is institutionally required in planning and implementing some public policies with a caring and respectful neuroscientific attitude towards the mind of particular human beings who happen to be subjects of scientific experiments. The results presented above will guide us in asking which are the fairest public policies and institutions based on knowing-how to respect in a caring manner. The use of drugs to treat students is morally required given the above considerations, but a particular state may also have other priorities based on justice. It seems also clear that the state must beforehand have, in society's name, sound guidelines for the public use of stimulants for adults, for instance, by regulating the participation and potential abuses of the pharmaceutical industry.

One of the first public policies necessary is to include neurobioethical issues to the educational system itself. In this sense, we can use the existing proposals for teaching bioethics and simply add more ethical questions related to the mind and brain. Bioethics is part of the curriculum for many health professionals, including proposals for teaching responsibilities.[73] Besides, bioethics already has a set of working institutions (e.g., the IRBs already mentioned in the previous chapter) at many levels. Here we see that neuro*bioethics* has a great advantage over neuroethics since the latter has not been fully institutionlized yet. Thus, it would not be a too difficult to deal with moral issues surrounding the mind in the classroom.

The results of the previous section were clear in the sense that existing cognitive enhancers must not be used by healthy students since they affect the neurodevelopment of the PFC, lead to addiction, etc. Now, even a diagnosis of ADHD must be made with great care. Later in life, the person may struggle with other mental disorders, for instance become anxious, depressed, etc. Thus, I would now like to say a few words on how caring respect may work in psychiatry in general. Many medical areas need to improve care in the direction of respecting persons more and not seeing patients as clients to be treated only, but psychiatry is one of the mostcritical given the increasing incidence of "modern" disorders such as anxiety, depression, etc. It is said that "Psychiatrists remain the only medical

[73] For instance, the United Nations has many important recommendations on this point: http://www.unesco.org/new/en/social-and-human-sciences/themes/bioethics/

specialist that never look at the organ they treat." (*Apud* Farah and Gillihan 2013, 128). Now, an accurate diagnosis is an ethical imperative in medicine in general and in psychiatry in particular. Thus, how can we then improve the diagnosis of mental disorders? Farah and Gillihan have discussed the potential benefits and the limits of neuroimaging in clinical psychiatry, arguing that there are reasons to expect the diagnostic system will change towards incorporating more imaging data.[74] This appears to be a welcome development because diagnoses in psychiatry are still mainly based on behavioral criteria: "We diagnose depression by asking the patient how he feels and whether his sleeping, eating, and other behaviors have changed. We diagnose attention deficit hyperactivity disorder (ADHD) by asking the patient, family member, and others about the patient's tendency to get distracted, act impulsively, and so on." (Farah and Gillihan 2013, 128). Now, one of the main problems is that many psychiatrists quickly (over)diagnose a mental disorder or a dysfunction in the neurotransmitters and start prescribing drugs without due care, disrespecting the patient as a person.

To overcome this state of affairs we need new conceptual investigations as well as more empirical research. For instance, what does it mean to say that a patient suffers from a mental disorder? To start answering this question, consider how the APA (American Psychiatric Association) changed the definition of mental disorder from DSM-IV to DSM-V. First, it was stated:

> A mental disorder is a clinically significant behavioral or psychological syndrome or pattern that occurs in an individual and that is associated with present distress or disability or with a significantly increased risk of suffering death, pain, disability, or an important loss of freedom. (DSM-IV, 2000)

That was, really, too vague. Much can fit under this broad definition. After all, what does it mean to say that a person has "a significantly increased risk of suffering" from "loss of freedom"? Thus, it was redefined in the newly released APA document in these terms:

> A mental disorder is a syndrome characterized by clinically significant disturbance in an individual'scognition,emotion regulation, or behavior that reflects a dysfunction in the psychological, biological, or developmental processes underlying mental functioning. (DSM-V, 2013)

---

[74] The use of biomarkers for diagnoses in psychiatry is defended by Baum (2016, 26).

There is no doubt that this is a better definition. Neuroscience played a huge role in establishing a more reliable and clinically significant classification of mental disorders based on neural dysfunctions, but it remains unclear whether its till allows for too much.

Aware of this problem, the definition is supplemented with warnings, namely that mental disorders should be associated with *significant distress*. Granted, according to the APA, a culturally approved response to a *common stressor* or loss such as the death of a loved one is not a mental disorder. In the same vein, socially deviant behavior (e.g., political, religious, or sexual) and conflicts that are primarily between the individual and society are not mental disorders unless the deviance results from a *dysfunction* in the individual. I remain, however, a bit skeptical as to whether the APA has found a better way to avoid overdiagnosis and overmedicalization in the psychiatric field. Granted, the DSM-V makes no prognosis, but it is still open to considering almost any symptom of sadness, or even a worry, to be medicalized, which may lead to fraudulent practices indeed. Should a melancholic mood be medically treated or just assumed as a human existential trait? Should it be considered a *common stressor* or is it clearly a *dysfunction*? It may well be an existential condition for art, philosophy, etc. I do not mean to imply that most mental disorders are not dysfunctions or impairments, but a so-wide definition as to include *distress* opens the door to identifying non-existent unhealthy conditions.

To argue for this point, I would now like to compare briefly what is going on in the diagnosis of ADHD with some other psychiatric conditions as they are stated in the DSM-V. Consider, firstly, schizophrenia. According to the APA, as a psychotic disorder, it has to be identified by abnormalities in one or more of the following five domains: delusions, hallucinations, disorganized thinking (speech), grossly disorganized or abnormal motor behavior (including catatonia), and negative symptoms. All these are *signs* (not only symptoms) and can clearly be empirically *verified.* But consider, secondly, bipolar and its related disorders. In the DSM-V, they were separated from the depressive disorders, and the diagnoses include bipolar I disorder, bipolar II disorder, cyclothymic disorder, substance/medication-induced bipolar and related disorder and unspecified bipolar and related disorder. Here, it is already *less clear* what, for instance, "unspecified bipolar and related disorder" is meant to be. Now, consider, thirdly, depressive disorders themselves: they include disruptive mood dysregulation disorder, major depressive disorder (including major depressive episodes), persistent depressive disorder (dysthymia), premenstrual dysphoric disorder, substance/medication-induced depressive disorderand, again, unspecified depressive disorder. The common feature of all of these disorders is the presence of a sad, empty, or irritable mood, accompanied by somatic and cognitive changes that significantly affect the individual's capacity to function. What differs among them are issues of duration, timing, or presumed etiology. At this point, *it is just not clear* whether a "sad, empty, or irritable mood" is really a disorder needing treatment, even if it causes some distress as melancholy does.[75] The diagnoses of these disorders may be made on *symptoms* only, not necessarily on clear *signs*. Fourthly, consider also how the DSM-V describes anxiety disorders: they include disorders that share features of excessive fear and anxiety and related behavioral disturbances. The definitions of "fear" and "anxiety" are plain enough: fear is the emotional response to real or perceived imminent threat; anxiety is the anticipation of a future threat. Once again, the diagnoses of these disorders may be made on *symptoms* only, not necessarily on empirically verifiable *signs*. Finally, panic attacks feature within the anxiety disorders as a particular type of fear response. Now, we may ask: are anxiety and panic attacks always in need of pharmacological treatment? *Clearly*, the answer is "No!" There are many techniques to deal with them besides the prevalent biomedical model.

We need both more acute conceptual analyses and more empirical research in psychiatry. Above all, however, caring respect is urgently required. What do we mean when we say that a mental condition, such as adolescent antisocial behavior, sadness, intense worry, panic, shyness, etc. is not merely a form of normal, human functioning, but indicative of a psychiatric disorder? Psychiatry's credibility, as a medical field, depends on a convincing answer to such questions. Some distressing conditions need not be medicalized. There are different ways of dealing with shyness without appealing to drugs. A good starting point is, perhaps, to make the distinction between *value* (*ethical*) and *factual* (scientific) elements. It is time to recognize that many psychiatric concepts have normative ingredients based on value judgements. Thus, they are not biomedical terms only, but include sociopolitical conditions. One should, on one hand, bear in mind that a disorder is a dysfunction and *dysfunction* is a scientific factual term, referring to a failure of biologically designed functioning. On the other hand, "harm" is most of the time a value term referring to conditions judged negatively by sociocultural standards. That is to say, there are harmful stresses and unharmful ones. Consequently, we cannot so quickly jump,

---

[75] It is worth pointing out that since the first DSM, back in 1952, the APA's catalogue went from 106 disorders to almost 300 in the DSM-V. This is a bit worrying since psychiatric diagnosis must be driven by evidence-based research and not by other interests, for instance pharmaceutical companies' earnings and profits. Rightly, the British Psychological Society has expressed concerns regarding DSM-V.

without further explanation, from a *distress* to a *disorder* and then to treatment.

It is too easy in psychiatry to go from the diagnosis of panic, through a supposed anxiety problem, to the prognosis and treatment for some kind of depression. Now, a *caring* respectful psychiatrist avoids overdiagnosis and the medicalization of life. Panic cannot obviously be underestimated but need also not be overdiagnosed: first of all, one needs to learn how to calm down, to control, to breathe ... Maybe it is due to something that should not actually bother us. In some cases, there is no need to medicalize, that is, to define the problem in medical termsor use a medical intervention to treat it. The same applies to some cases of "attention deficit" or even "hyperactivity." Thus, a caring respectful person is well aware of the perils of overdiagnosis and the medicalization of life driven by the huge interests of the big pharmaceutical companies.

I believe that, nowadays, both overdiagnosis and excessive medicalization result in more people receiving unjustifiable medical treatment. Medicalization of life is created by a specific set of cultural and social conditions, and can be propelled by forces outside medicine, especially by the industry.[76] Recalling the case presented at the beginning of the previous section, it may start with some perception of anxious behavior as presented by many teens in school who are then too rapidly sent to counseling resulting in treatment for a psychiatric disorder. Once again, society as a whole has to take more care in many *experimental* treatments in psychiatry: what are we doing to our kids by allowing them to switch from one drug to another; to take combinations of drugs; to progress to more and more new "modern" drugs, which are supposedly safer and more efficient? If we allow the pharmaceutical industry and doctors who prescribe "one too many" drugs to go ahead, then society itself will end up dysfuncional. This is the opposite of what neurobio*ethics*, based on caring respect, is all about. The suggestion, then, in institutional terms, is that the educational system must work in the direction of *preventing* the use of drugs, not encouraging students to take them to enhance their performance.

Other institutional arrangements are, however, essential to prevent overdiagnosis and overmedicalization on a large scale. What are, then, the best public policies to manage mental disorders such as ADHD in teenagers based on caring respect and, perhaps in the future, safe and efficient cognitive enhancers for adults? To begin to answer this question, I would like to examine some proposals already made on this issue. In their

[76] For an official recommendation to be more cautious when prescribing smart drugs see: American Academy of Neurology at
https://www.aan.com/PressRoom/Home/PressRelease/1163

contribution to *The Oxford Handbook of Neuroethics*, Thomas Metzinger and Elisabeth Hildt sorted out, in chapter 15 entitled "Cognitive Enhancement", some suggestions, and I would simply like to restate them here: (i) the role of medicine and the aims of medicine are of central relevance in so far as they serve as a *legitimization* for a certain procedure, introducing new neurotechnologies into society;[77] (ii) governments, medical associations, and other professional organizations in the field of medicine are obliged to *actively monitor* the process in which medical taxonomies, diagnosis manuals, etc. continuously evolve; (iii) policy makers should stay clear of ideological debates; (iv) all decisions must be evidence-based; (v) it is necessary to thoroughly and *objectively* inform the public on the effects, side effects, chances, and risks of cognition-enhancing substances; (vi) all forms of direct-to-customer marketing should be prohibited;[78] (vii) policy making cannot be confined to devising new regulations. There are other suggestions, but these are the most important in helping us grasp the responsibilities of the state to treat mental disorders and eventually legislate on cognitive enhancers. I would like to emphasize the first two, namely the special role of medicine and medical associations and other similar organizations in the healthcare sector to guarantee that caring respect, as defined in the last chapter, is really in place in such programs.

Another institutional arrangement relates to the need for a fairer healthcare system. I will now defend a Rawlsian proposal which is an implication of applying practical cognitivism and the first principle of ethics leading to the fundamental concept of caring respect. As we have seen in this work, a particular material criterion of justice is required by neurobioethics, namely to treat each person according to her basic needs. Now, Rawls himself came, as it is perhaps well known, to recognize that priority must be given to such a criterion. In his own words, a norm

> (...) covering the equal basic rights and liberties may easily be preceded by a lexically prior principle requiring that *citizen's basic needs* been met, at least insofar as their being met is necessary for citizens to understand and to be able fruitfully to exercise those rights and liberties. (1993, 7, italics added)

---

[77] In her work "The Case for Clinical Management of Neuroenhancement in Young People," Ilina Singh agrees on this point: "In our view, it is imperative to locate a relevant site where US young people's uses of neuroenhancement technologies can be safely, objectively, and ethically evaluated and managed. *We propose that this site should be the primary care clinic*." (Singh 2013, 26-27, italics added)

[78] Direct-to-consumer advertising is prohibited in all countries, except the United States and New Zealand.

As can be seen, the right to a fair go may not be the most basic principle in terms of distributive justice. Anyway, the prioritization of the satisfaction of basic needs over other rights is fully supported by the first principle of ethics; namely, it is optimific, universally willable and would not be rejected by a virtuous person.

Rawls agrees in his late work that the satisfaction of basic needs has priority over the classical liberal principle of basic liberties, which in turn, were prioritized above social and economic inequalities that needed to be arranged so that they were both (i) to everyone's interest, especially to the greatest benefit of those least advantaged, and (ii) attached to offices and positions open to all under conditions of fair equality of opportunity. Thus, a right to a fair go needs to be preceded by a right to have basic needs satisfied. This is what caring respect requires too, and this is justified by the first principle of ethics.

There is no space of course to discuss all the socially required arrangements for neurobioethics. Thus, I would here like to mention at least one more institution I believe is necessary to implement effectively distributive justice regarding drugs such as amphetamine, namely a *mixed* universal healthcare system, which is neither what we happen to have in Brazil and UK (universal coverage) nor the US (based on insurance only) at the moment. On this point, I would like to quote a Rawlsian-inspired institution defended by the bioethicists Beauchamp and Childress. A mixed system would comprise two tiers:

> **First tier**: enforced social coverage for basic and catastrophic health needs (public health protection and preventive care, primary care, acute care, and special social services for those with disabilities), that is, universal access to basic services.
>
> …
>
> **Second tier**: private coverage for other health needs and desires (luxury hospital rooms and optional, cosmetic dental work etc.) available for purchase at personal expense through private health insurance or direct payment. (Beauchamp & Childress 2013, 273)

Note that the first tier covers basic health needs such as treatment for ADHD. Similar proposals based on a Rawlsian conception of justice as fairness have also been made by Norman Daniels (1995, 2008) using the fair opportunity principle and have the potential to reach an overlapping consensus. Granted, giving priority to the worst-off is not something most deontologists, consequentialists and virtue ethicists would disagree with. Thus, I will now argue for a person-centered health care system based on such an assumption and as a requirement to institutionalize caring respect.

One way of overcoming the abusive use of drugs towards a more caring respectful attitude in neurobioethics can perhaps be grasped in what is sometimes referred to as "patient-centered care." As it is well-known, this movement began more than two decades ago and was embraced by governments (US, UK etc.), healthcare providers and insurance companies.[79] It means that providers, patients and families work together to provide better healthcare for the patient.[80] There are two steps to providing patient-centered care:

i) patients and their families actively participate in their own healthcare by sharing their own needs and preferences;
ii) providers listen to these needs, and then focus their education and training on ensuring better healthcare outcomes.

Thus, patient-centered care seems respectful as previously defined in this work: it respects *you* as a whole person, *your* right to assistance, but also to privacy etc. In turn, the patient must respect the healthteam as partners in caring. When decisions about care are shared, it is respectful indeed.

Despite the fact that a precise definition of "person-centered care" is difficult to offer, some believe that it is based on four principles: (i) affording people dignity, compassion and respect; (ii) offering coordinated care; (iii) offering personalized care, support or treatment; (iv) supporting people to recognize and develop their own strengths and abilities to enable them to live independent and fulfilling lives. What are the similarities and differences between caring respect/respectful care and person-centered care? From the theoretical point of view, they look very similar since both are, for instance, based on moral sentiments (sympathy, compassion) and on respect.[81] Is it not clear, however, whether patient-centered care requires an *intrinsic valuation* of the person, as I have argued for in this book,

---

[79] For the theoretical bases of a patient-centered medicine see: Stewart (2014). The Health Foundation published, in 2104, a quick guide called "Person-centered care made simple":
https://www.health.org.uk/sites/health/files/PersonCentredCareMadeSimple.pdf.
Information of the movement can be found here:
https://www.ncbi.nlm.nih.gov/pubmed/24696963

[80] In Brazil, a similar movement, the so-called "HumanizaSUS," began back in 2003, focusing on a more respectful caring attitude. More information can be found here (in Portuguese): http://bvsms.saude.gov.br/bvs/humanizacao/pub_destaques.php

[81] Another similarity is the integral approach since in person-centered care "we use the word 'person' in order to emphasize a holistic approach to care, that takes into account the whole person – not a narrow focus on their condition or symptoms but also their preferences, well-being and wider social and cultural background."

expecting also from the patient herself an attitude of self-care and self-respect. To compare these two approaches to care is, however, not the main purpose of this work.

To finish this section, I would like to synthesize what I have done in this last chapter. I have discussed whether neuroscience brings new ethical challenges which cannot be dealt with using the the concept of caring respect previously defended. To avoid empty generalizations, I have discussed non-conventional cognitive enhancement, which seems to have benefits, but we must beware abuses— cheating, addiction, compromising juvenile brain development, false promises by the pharmaceutical industry and so on. Knowing-how to respect a person in a caring manner leads, then, to the following conclusion: cognitive non-conventional enhancers are not morally permissible for young students because they affect the PFC's plasticity. It does not follow, however, that a safe and efficient enhancer cannot be used by adults. This, in turn, creates issues around social justice. Now, since there are other public urgencies (e.g. relieving misery so children's brains grow healthily), then the state must give priority to these policies instead of focusing on positive cognitive enhancement, although it coud, if safe and efficient, be sought through private means. The main conclusion, then, is that a practical cognitivist would recommend avoiding the prescription of neuroenhancing drugs for children and adolescents in contexts where it may not be *for their own sake*, for instance, because of parent's or school's expectations. The person (the patient, the subject of neuroscientific research and experiments) *herself* must be the center of caring respect.

FINAL REMARKS

In this book, I worked out a new moral epistemology based on the thesis that moral knowledge involves knowing-how in order to provide support to the concept of *caring respect* as a basic ingredient of *a* CS-Morality and applied it to neurobioethical issues, especially cognitive enhancement. The main point was to sort out the argument that we need practical cognitivism to overcome the main problems of the intuitionist meta-ethics of the predominant bioethical theory and to make caregivers recognize that proper caring respect requires a special kind of knowledge, not only technical knowing-how, but explicit moral knowing-how: namely, valuing intrinsically the cared for including human subjects of scientific experiments. Thus, knowing-how to respect in a caring manner is most needed in bioethics (and in neuroethics as well) to avoid negligence and to provide the best possible care for potential subjects of neuroscientific research and its neurotechnological applications, for instance using experimental drugs to boost cognitive performance.

To accomplish these goals, I have argued for three main ideas: (i) that *neuro*ethics, understood as the neuroscience of morality, is a scientific study among others and that one cannot consider it normative *ethics* because this would be a category mistake; (ii) that neuro*ethics*, taken to be the ethics of neuroscience, is best understood as neurobio*ethics*, a specific subfield of applied ethics; therefore, (iii) that the best normative framework for neuroscientific investigations using human beings is provided by the *Belmont Report* based on respect for persons and not for individual autonomy only, which makes sense of public policies leading to a person-centered healthcare system and so on.

This result also gives support to the main warning in *Nature Neuroscience*, namely that neuroscientists doing scientific research and experiments using human subjects must be held accountable if they violate the basic rights of the person such as mental privacy. Only neurobio*ethics*, not the supposedly "new field" of *neuro*ethics, shows that they cannot evade responsibility. This is one of the main results of this work. The conclusion, then, is that we need to support the *Nature* editorial's call: the ethical neuroscientist must follow the Belmont guidelines not only in academic institutions but in the private sector too! Respect for persons do not require new laws to protect vulnerable populations from neuroscientific and neurotechnological potential abuses, but better practices only.

Last but not least, I would like to go back to one of the main neuroethics challenges, namely how to avoid the growing role of neuroscience in society as a whole lapsing into nihilism. I hope to have presented a sound argument to refute the view that personhood is just an illusion. Moreover, I have argued that the principle of respect for persons is well grounded on the first principle of ethics. Thus, it must be fully observed in states governed by the rule of law and implemented in our everyday practices, leading to attitudes such as *caring respect*. It may also make us rethink some of our institutions, for instance towards a fairer person-centred healthcare system. It can then provide caring respect in a personalized way following a holistic approach and not only evidence-based medicine guided exclusively by the biomedical predominant paradigm. This means that, among other things, most medical areas, especially psychiatry, need to put the person before the subject of research or the patient. This avoids the neurosciences reducing persons to machices. That would be against one of the most basic moral requirementsof neurobio*ethics*.

REFERENCES

American Psychiatric Association. *Diagnostic and Statistical Manual of Mental Disorders: DSM-5*. Arlington, 2013.

Araújo, M. Moral Enhancement and Political Realism. *Journal of Evolution and Technology*. V.24, 2014, pp.29-43.

Aristotle. *Nicomachean Ethics* (trans. by Roger Crisp). Cambridge: Cambridge University Press, 2014.

Arrington, R. A Wittgensteinian Approach to Ethical Intuitionism. In: Stratton-Lake, Philip (ed.). *Ethical Intuitionism: Re-evaluations*. Oxford: Clarendon Press, 2002. pp.271-289.

Audi, R. *The Good in the Right*. A theory of Intuition and Intrinsic Value. New Jersey: Princeton University Press, 2004.

Azevedo, M. A. Health as a Clinic-Epidemilogical Concept. *Journal of Evaluation in Clinical Practice*. 21(3), 2015. pp. 265-73.

Azevedo, M. A. & Andrade, B. Tying Care and Respect into a Single Bioethical Principle: On Dall'Agnol's respectful care theory. *Journal of Evaluation in Clinical Practice*. May 2019. pp.1-6. https://doi.org/10.1111/jep.13150

Baker, G. & Hacker, P. *Wittgenstein Rules, Grammar and Necessity*. Oxford: Wiley Blackwell, 2014.

Bakhurst, D. Minds, Brains and Education. *Journal of Philosophy of Education*. Vol. 42, No. 3-4, 2008

Barros, D. B. As representações sociais do uso do metilfenidato: do tratamento ao aprimoramento cognitivo. Rio de Janeiro: Tese de Doutorado (UERJ), 2014.

Baum, M. L. *The Neuroethics of Biomarkers*. What the Development of Bioprediction Means for Moral Responsibility, Justice, and the Nature of Mental Disorder. Oxford: Oxford University Press, 2016.

Bear, M. R. & Connors, B. & Paradiso, M. A. *Neuroscience. Exploring the Brain.* (4ed.) Philadelphia: Wolters Kluwer, 2016.

Beauchamp, T. & Childress, J. *Principles of Biomedical Ethics*(7ªed.). Oxford: University Press, 2013.

Bengson, J.& Moffett, M. (eds). *Knowing how: Essays on Knowledge, Mind, and Action*. Oxford: Oxford University Press, 2012.

Bennett, M.R. & Hacker, P.M.S. *Philosophical Foundations of Neuroscience*. Oxford: Blackwell, 2010.

Bennett, M. R. & Dennett, D. & Hacker, P.M.S. & Searle, J. *Neuroscience and Philosophy: Brain, Mind, and Language*. With an Introduction and Conclusion by Daniel Robinson. New York: Columbia University Press, 2007.

Bentham, J. *The Principles of Morals and Legislation.* New York: Hafner Press, 1948.

Black, D. B. & Andreasen, N. C. *Introductory Textbook of Paychiatry*. Washington/London: American Psychiatirc Publishing, 2014

Blackburn, S. Reply: Rule-Following and Moral Realism. In: Holzman, S. &Leich, C. *Wittgenstein: to follow a rule*. London: Routledge: 1981. pp.163-187.

Blackburn, Simon. *Essays in Quasi-Realism*. New York/Oxford: Oxford University Press, 1993.

Borém, Aluízio *et al. Understanding Biotechnology*. Upper Saddle River, Prentice Hall, 2003.

Borenstein, J.& Pearson, Y. Robot Caregivers: Ethical Issues across the Human Lifespan. In: Lin, Patrick *et al.* (eds). *Robot Ethics*. *The Ethical and Social Implications of Robotics*. Cambridge, Mass./London: The MIT Press, 2012. pp.251-265.

Bostrom, N. & Roache, R. Smart Policy: Cognitive Enhancement and the Public Interest. In: Savulescu, Julian *et al.* (eds.). *Enhancing Human Capacities*. Oxford: Oxford University Press, 2011. pp.138-149.

Brandt, R. *Morality, Utilitarianism and Rights*. New York: Cambridge, Cambridge University Press, 1992.

Buchman, A. *Beyond Humanity*? Oxford: Oxford University Press, 2013.

Cabrera, L. Environmental Neuroethics: Setting the Foundations. In: Illes, J. (ed.) *Neuroethics*. *Anticipating the Future*.Oxford: Oxford University Press, 2017.p. 426-454.

Callahan, D. Bioethics as a Discipline. In: Jecker, N.*et al*. (eds). *Bioethics*. *An Introduction to the History, Methods, and Practice.* Sudbury: Jones and Bartlett Publishers, 1997. pp.17-22.

Caplan, A. *et al.* (eds.) *The Case of Terri Schiavo*. *Ethics at the End of Life*. New York: Prometheus Books, 2006.

Carter, R. *Mapping the Mind*. London: Weidenfeld & Nicolson, 2010.

Chancellor, B. & Chatterjee, A. Brain Training. In: Chatterjee, A. & Farah, M. *Neuroethics in Practice. Medicine, Mind, and Society.* Oxford: Oxford University Press, 2013. pp.57-66.

Chatterjee, A. Brain Enhancement in Healthy Adults. In: Chatterjee, A. & Farah, M. *Neuroethics in Practice. Medicine, Mind, and Society.* Oxford: Oxford University Press, 2013. pp.3-15

Chatterjee, A. & Farah, M. *Neuroethics in Practice. Medicine, Mind, and Society.* Oxford: Oxford University Press, 2013.

Charon, R.& Montello, M. (eds.). *Stories Matter. The Role of Narrative in Medical Ethics*. New York/London: Routledge, 2002.

Chen, D. &Quirion, R. From the Internationalization to the Globalization of Neuroethics: Some Perspectives and Challenges. In: Illes, J. & Sahakian, B. (eds). *The Oxford Handbook of Neuroethics*. Oxford: Oxford University Press, 2013. pp. 823-834.

Childress, J.*et al.* (eds). *Belmont Revisited. Ethical Principles for Research with Human Subjects*. Washington: Georgetown University Press, 2005.

Chomsky, N. *Rules and Representations*. New Youk: Columbia University Press, 1980.

Churchland, P. *Neurophilosophy*. Camb./MA: Cambridge University Press, 1989.

Clark, A. and Chalmers, D. The Extended Mind. *Analysis*. (58), 1998. pp.7-19.

Cortina, A. *Neuroética y Neuropolítica*. Sugerencias para la educacíon moral. Madrid: Tecnos, 2018.

Conrad, E. C. & de Vries, R. Field of Dreams: A Social History of Bioethics. *Advances in Medical Sociology*. (13), 2011. pp. 299-324.

Crick, F. *The Astonishing Hypothesis*. London: Touchstone, 1995.

Crisp, R. Treatment According to Need: Justice and the British National Health Service. In: Rhodes, Rosamond *et al.* (eds.) *Medicine and Social Justice. Essays on the Distribution of Health Care*. Oxford: Oxford University Press, 2002. pp. 134-143.

Crisp, R. Equality, Priority, and Compassion. *Ethics*. 113(4), pp.754-763.

Crisp, R. *Reasons & the Good.* Oxford: Oxford University Press, 2006.

Crisp, R. *Griffin on Human Rights.* Oxford: Oxford University Press, 2014.

Crisp, R. & Dall'Agnol, D. & Tonetto, M. C. & Savulescu, J. (orgs) *Ética Aplicada e Políticas Públicas*. Florianópolis: Edufsc, 2018.

Cummiskey, D. *Kantian Consequentialism*. Oxford: Oxford University Press, 2003.

Dall'Agnol, D. Respect for persons. Rawls' Kantian Principles. In: Dall'Agnol, D. & Tonetto, M. *Morality and Life. Kantian Perspectives in Bioethics*. Pisa: ETS, 2015a. pp.127-145.

Dall'Agnol, D. Practical Cognitivism: Knowing-how to Follow a Moral Rule. In: Kanzian, C.*et al.* (eds) *Realism, Relativism and Constructivism.* Kichberg am Wechsel: WAB archives, 2015b. pp.53-55.

Dall'Agnol, D. Knowing-how to care. *Journal of Medical Ethics*, v.42 (3). 2016a. pp. 1-6.

Dall'Agnol, D. *Care and Respect in Bioethics*. Newcastle: Cambridge Scholars, 2016b.

Dall'Agnol, D. *La ética en Wittgenstein y el problema del relativismo*. València: Publicacions de la Universitat de València, 2016c.

Dall'Agnol, D. Respect in Kant's *Tugendlehre* and its place in contemporary ethics. *ethic@*. Vol. 16, 2017. pp. 437-458.

Dall'Agnol, D. Ética y escepticismo en Wittgenstein. In: David Perez Chico. (Org.). Wittgenstein y el Escepticismo: Certeza, paradoxa y locura. Zaragoza: Prensas de La Universidad de Zaragoza, 2018. pp. 261-282.

Dall'Agnol, D. & de Azevedo, M.A.O. An agency model of consent and the standards of disclosure in health care: knowing-how to reach respectful shared decisions among real persons. *Journal of Evaluation in Clinical Practice*. 2019, pp.1-8. DOI: 10.1111/jep.13281

Damasio, A. R. *Descarte's Error: Emotion, Reason, and the Human Brain.* New York: G.P. Putnam, 1994.

Daniels, N. *Just Health Care.* Cambridge: Cambridge University Press, 1995.

Daniels, N. *Just health: Meeting Health Needs Fairly*. New York: Cambridge University Press, 2008.

Darwall, S. Two Kinds of Respect. *Ethics*.V.88. 1978. pp.36-49.

Darwall, S. *Philosophical Ethics*. Boulder: Westview Press, 1998.

Darwall, S. *Welfare and Rational Care.* Princeton/Oxford: Princeton University Press, 2004.

Darwall, S. *The Second-person Standpoint. Morality, Respect and Accountability.* Cambridge/London: Harvard University Press, 2006.

Darwin, C. *From So Simple a Beginning: the four great books of Charles Darwin*. New York/London: W. W. Norton & Company, 2006.

Dawkins, R. *The God Delusion*. Boston/New York: Houghton Mifflin Company: 2006.

De Dreu, C. *et al*. Oxytocin promotes human ethnocentrism. *Proceedings of the National Academy of Sciences*. 108(4), 2001, pp. 1262-1266.

Devall, B.& Sessions, G. Deep Ecology. In: Sterba, J. *Earth Ethics. Introductory Readings on Animal Rights and Environmental Ethics*. New Jersey: Prentice Hall, 2000. pp.149-157.

Diller, L. H. The Run on Ritalin: Attention Deficit Disorder and Stimulant Treatment in the 1990s. In: Farah, M. J. (ed.) *Neuroethics. An Introduction, with Readings.* Camb./MA: MIT Press, 2010. Pp.42-57

Dillon, R. Respect and Care: Toward Moral Integration. *Canadian Journal of Philosophy*. (22)1, 1992. pp. 105-132.

Dodge, T. & Williams, KJ. &Marzell, M. &Turrisi, R. Judging Cheaters: Is Substance Misuse Viewed Similarly in the Athletic and Academic Domains? Psychology of Addictive Behaviors. 2012, Vol. 26, No. 3, 678 – 682

dos Anjos, M. F. & Siqueira, J. E. (orgs.) *Bioética no Brasil. Tendências e perspectivas*. São Paulo: SBB/Idéias e Letras, 2007

Downie, R. S. & Telfer, E. *Respect for persons*. New York: Schocken Books, 1970.

Downie, R. S. &Calman, K. *Healthy Respect. Ethics in Health Care*. Oxford/New York: Oxford University Press, 1994.

Dworkin, R. *Taking Rights Seriously*. London: Duckworth, 1977.

Dworkin, R. *Life's Dominion. An Argument about Abortion, Euthanasia, and Individual Freedom.* New York: Alfred A. Knopf, 1993.

Dworkin, R. *Justice for Hedgehogs*. Cam./Mass & London: Harvard University Press, 2011.

Elliott, C. (ed.) *Slow Cures and Bad Philosophers. Essays on Wittgenstein, Medicine and Bioethics*. Durham/London: Duke University Press, 2001.

Elliot, C. Prozac as a Way of Life. In: Farah, M. J. (ed.) *Neuroethics. An Introduction, with Readings.* Camb./MA: MIT Press, 2010. pp.119-130

Emanuel, E. The Beginning of the End of Principlism. *Hastings Center Report*. N.25. 1995. pp.37-8.

Engelhardt, T. Ethical Issues in Aiding the Dearth of Young Children. In: Baird, R. & Rosembaum, S. (eds). *Euthanasia: The Moral Issues*. Buffalo: Prometheus Books, 1989. pp. 141-154.

Engelhardt, T. *The Foundations of Bioethics* (2ªed.). Oxford: Oxford University Press, 1996.

Engelhardt, T. (ed.). *Global Bioethics. The Collapse of Consensus*. Salem: MM Scrivener Press, 2006.

Engelhardt, T.&Jotterand, F. (eds.). *The Philosophy of Medicine Reborn: a Pellegrino Reader*. Notre Dame: University of Notre Dame Press, 2008.

Engster, D. *The Heart of Justice: Care Ethics and Political Theory*. Oxford: Oxford University Press, 2009.

Farah, M. J. Emerging Ethical Issues in Neuroscience. *Nature Neuroscience*. 5(11), 2002.

Farah, M. J. (ed.) *Neuroethics. An Introduction, with Readings.* Camb./MA: MIT Press, 2010.

Farah, M. J. &Heverlein, A. S. Personhood: An Illusion Rooted in Brain Function? In: Farah, M.J. (ed.) *Neuroethics. An Introduction, with Readings.* Camb./MA: MIT Press, 2010. pp. 321-338.

Farah, M. J. &Gillihan, S. Neuroimaging in Clinical Psychiatry. In: Chatterjee, A. & Farah, S. *Neuroethics in Practice. Medicine, Mind, and Society.* Oxford: Oxford University Press, 2013. pp.128-146.

Farah, M.J. Personhood, Consciousness, and Severe Brain Damage. In: Chatterjee, A. & Farah, S. *Neuroethics in Practice. Medicine, Mind, and Society.* Oxford: Oxford University Press, 2013. pp. 175-208.

Farah, M. Neuroscience and Neuroethics in the 21th Century. In: Illes, J. & Sahakian. (eds). *The Oxford Handbook of Neuroethics*. Oxford: Oxford University Press, 2013. pp.761-781.

Fins, J. J. & Schiff, N. D. Disorders of Counsciousness Following Severe Brain Injury. Chatterjee, A. & Farah, M. *Neuroethics in Practice. Medicine, Mind, and Society.* Oxford: Oxford University Press, 2013. pp.162-174.

Fuchs, T. Ethical Issues in Neuroscience. *Current Opinion in Psychiatry.* (19), 2006, pp. 600-7.

Gabriel, M. *I am not a Brain. Philosophy of Mind for the Twenty-first Century.* Cambridge: Polity Press, 2017.

Garrafa, V. &Pessini, L. *Bioética: Poder e Injustiça*. São Paulo: Loyola/São Camilo, 2004.

Gert, B.& Culver, C.&Clouser, D. *Bioethics. A Return to Fundamentals.* New York/Oxford: Oxford University Press, 1997.

Gibbard, A. *Wise Choices, Apt Feelings*. A Theory of Normative Judgment. Camb./Mass.: Harvard University Pres, 1992.

Gilligan, C. *In a Different Voice. Phychological Theory and Women's Development.* Massachusetts: Harvard University Press, 2003.

Glock, H.J. *A Wittgenstein Dictionary*. Oxford: Blackwell, 2005.

Greene, J. D. *et al.* An fMRI Investigation of Emotional Engagement in Moral Judgment. *Science*. Vol. 293, Sep 2001. pp. 2105-2018.

Greene, J. *Moral Tribes. Emotion, Reason, and the Gap Between Us and Them.* New York: Penguin, 2013.

Greene, J. & Cohen, J. For the Law, Neuroscience Changes Nothing and Everything. In: Illes, J. & Sahakian. (eds). *The Oxford Handbook of Neuroethics*. Oxford: Oxford University Press, 2013. pp.655-674

Greene, J. D. The Rat-a-gorical Imperative: Moral Intuition and the Limits of Affective Learning. *Cognition*, 2017 (In press).

Griffin, J. *On Human Rights*. Oxford: Oxford University Press, 2013.

Grosso, J. S. P. Desde la Bioética a la Neuro-ética: *Revista Latinoamericana de Bioética*. 13(2), 48-59, 2013.

Gyngell, C. & Douglas, T. & Savulescu, J. The Ethics of Germline Gene Editing. *Journal of Applied Philosophy*. November, 2016. DOI: 10.1111/japp.12249

Habermas, J. *Moral Consciousness and Communicative Action*. Camb./Mass., MIT Press, 1990.

Habermas, J. *The future of human nature*. Cambridge: Polity Press, 2003.

Hacker, P. *Insight and Illusion*. Themes in Philosophy of Wittgenstein. (Revised Edition) Oxford: Clarendon Press, 1986.

Hacker, P. *Wittgenstein's Place in Twentieth-century Analytic Philosophy*. Oxford: Blackwell, 1996.

Hacker, P. *Wittgenstein: Comparations &Context*. Oxford: Oxford University Press, 2013.

Hadskis, M. R. & Schmidt, M. H. Pediatric Neuroimaging Research. In: Illes, J. & Sahakian, B. (eds). *The Oxford Handbook of Neuroethics*. Oxford: Oxford University Press, 2013. pp.389-404.

Hare, R. *Moral Thinking: its Level, Methods, and Point*. Oxford: Oxford University Press, 1981.

Hare, R. Could Kant Have Been a Utilitarian? In: Hare, Richard. *Sorting Out Ethics*. Oxford: Clarendon Press, 2000.

Hare, R. *Essays on Bioethics*. Oxford: Clarendon Press, 2002.

Harris, J. Chemical Cognitive Enhancement: is it Unfair, Unjust, Discriminatory, or Cheating for Healthy Adults to Use Smart Drugs? In: Illes, J. & Sahakian, B. (eds). *The Oxford Handbook of Neuroethics*. Oxford: Oxford University Press, 2013. pp. 265-272.

Heidegger, M. *Being and Time*. New York: State University Of New York Press, 1996.

Held, V. *Justice and Care. Essential Readings in Feminist Ethics*. Colorado/Oxford: Westview Press, 1995.

Held, V. *The Ethics of Care. Personal, Political, and Global.* New York: Oxford University Press, 2006.

Hohfeld, W. N. *Fundamental Legal Conceptions as Applied in Judicial Reasoning and Other Legal Essays*. Yale University Press, 1919.

Hugher, J. Ultimate Justification: Wittgenstein and Medical Ethics. *Journal of Medical Ethics*, (21), 1995, pp.25-30.

Hume, D. *A Treatise on Human Nature*. Oxford: At Clarendon Pres, 1978.

Hume, D. *Enquires Concerning Human Understanding and Concerning the Principles of Morals*. Oxford: Clarendon Press, 1996.

Husserl, E. *The Idea of Phenomenology*. The Hague: MartinusNijhoff, 1973.

Hyman, S. E. Addiction and Responsibility. In: Chatterjee, A. & Farah, S. *Neuroethics in Practice. Medicine, Mind, and Society.* Oxford: Oxford University Press, 2013. pp.96-102.

Hyman, S. E. The Neurobiology of Addiction: Implications for Voluntary Control of Behavior. In: Illes, J. & Sahakian. (eds). *The Oxford*

Handbook of Neuroethics. Oxford: Oxford University Press, 2013. pp.203-217.

Illes, J. & Sahakian, B. (eds). *The Oxford Handbook of Neuroethics*. Oxford: Oxford University Press, 2013.

Illes, J. (ed.) *Neuroethics.Anticipating the Future*. Oxford: Oxford University Press, 2017.

Jahr, F. Bio-Ethics. In: Amir Muzur& Hans-Martin Sass (eds.) *Fritz Jahr and the Foundations of Global Bioethics*. Berlin: Lit Verlag, 2012. pp.1-4.

Jecker, N.*et al.* (eds.) *Bioethics. An Introduction to the History, Methods, and Practice*. Sudbury: Jones and Bartlett Publishers, 2007.

Johnson, L. *A Morally Deep World: An Essay on Moral Significance and Environmental Ethics*. Cambridge: Cambridge University Press, 1991.

Jonas, H. *The Imperative of Responsibility. In Search of an Ethics for the Technological Age*. Chicago: Chicago University Press, 1984.

Jonas, H. Philosophical Reflections on Experimenting with Human Subjects. In: Jecker, N.*et al.* (eds) *Bioethics. An Introduction to the History, Methods, and Practice*. Sudbury: Jones and Bartlett Publishers, 2007. pp. 44-52.

Jonsen, A. Do No Harm: Axiom of Medical Ethics. In: Spicker, S.& Engelhardt, T. *Philosophical and Medical Ethics: Its Nature and Significance*. Dordrecht: Reidel, 1977. pp. 27-41.

Jonsen, A. *The Birth of Bioethics*. New York/Oxford: Oxford University Press, 2003.

Jonsen, A. & Toulmin, S. *The Abuse of Casuistry. A History of Moral Reasoning*. Berkeley: University of California Press, 1988.

Kant, I. *Practical Philosophy*. Cambridge: Cambridge University Press, 2008.

Kant, I. *Werkausgabe* (edited by WihelmWeischedel). Frankfurt am Main, Surkamp, 1968.

Korsgaard, C. M. The Reasons We Can Share. An Attack on the Distinction between Agent-Relative and Agent-Neutral Value.*Social Philosophy and Policy*, 1993, 10(1).

Korsgaard, C. *Creating the Kingdom of Ends*. Cambridge: Cambridge University Press, 1996.

Kuhse, H.& Singer, P. (eds.) *Bioethics. An Anthology*. Oxford: Blackwell, 2006.

Kotulak, R. Teens Driven to Distraction. *Chicago Tribune*. March 24, 2006.

Kuusela, O.& McGinn, M. (eds.) *The Oxford Handbook of Wittgenstein*. Oxford: Oxford University Press, 2014.

Lantos, J.& Meadow, W. *Neonatal Bioethics. The Moral Challenges of Medical Innovation.* Baltimore: The Johns Hopkins University Press, 2006.

Leopold, A. The Land Ethic. In: Zimmerman, M.E. *et al. Environmental Philosophy.* From Animal Rights to Radical Ecology. New Jersey: Pearson Prentice Hall, 1993. pp. 102-115.

Levy, P. *Neuroethics.* New York/Cambridge: Cambridge University Press, 2007.

Levy, P. Neuroethics and the Extended Mind. In: Illes, J. & Sahakian. (eds). *The Oxford Handbook of Neuroethics.* Oxford: Oxford University Press, 2013. pp.285-294.

Libet, B. Unconscious Cerebral Initiative and the Role of Conscious Will in Voluntary Action. *Behavioral and Brain Sciences.* 8(4), 1985, pp.529-39.

Lindemann, H. *An Invitation to Feminist Ethics.* Boston: McGraw-Hill, 2006.

Little, M. Wittgensteinian Lessons on Moral Particularism. In: Elliott, Carl. (ed.) *Slow Cures and Bad Philosophers. Essays on Wittgenstein, Medicine and Bioethics.* Durham/London: Duke University Press, 2001. pp. 161-180.

Luciana, M. Development of the Adolescent Brain: Neuroethical Implications for the Understanding of Executive Function and Social Cognition. In: Illes, J. & Sahakian, B. *The Oxford Handbook of Neuroethics.* Oxford: Oxford University Press,2013. pp.59-82

MacIntyre, Ar. *After Virtue. A Study in Moral Theory.* London: Duckworth, 1994.

MacIntyre, A. *Whose Justice? Which Rationality.* London: Duckworth, 1988.

Mackie, J. L. *Ethics: inventing right and wrong.* London: Penguin, 1977.

Manson, N.& O'Neil, O. *Rethinking Informed Consent in Bioethics.* Cambridge: Cambridge University Press, 2007.

Maxwell, N. *From Knowledge to Wisdom. A Revolution for Science and the Humanities.* London: Pentire Press, 2007.

McGinn, M. &Kussela, O. *The Oxford Hanbook of Wittgenstein.* Oxford: Oxford University Press, 2014.

McNaughton, D. *The Moral Vision*: An Introduction to Ethics. Oxford: Basil Blackwell, 1988.

Medical Professionalism in the New Millennium: APhysician's Charter. *Medical Journal of Australia.* V. 177, 2002. pp.263-265.

Menary, T.(ed.) *The Extended Mind.* Cam.Mass./London: The MIT Press, 2010.

Metzinger, T. &Hildt, E. Cognitive Enhancement. In: Illes, J. & Sahakian, B. (eds). *The Oxford Handbook of Neuroethics*. Oxford: Oxford University Press, 2013. pp. 245-264.
Mill, J. S. *Utilitarianism*. Oxford: Oxford University Press, 2011.
Mill, J. S. *On Liberty and Other Writings*. Cambridge: Cambridge University Press, 1994.
Milner, B. *et al.* Cognitive Neuroscience and the Study of Memory. *Neuron*. (20)3, 1998, p.445-468.
Moll, J. *et al.* Frontopolar and Anterior Temporal Cortex Activation in a Moral Judgement Task. Preliminary functional MRI Results in Normal Subjects. *ArqNeuropsiquiatry*. 59(3-B), 2001, pp.657-664.
Moore, G. E. *Principia Ethica*. Cambridge: Cambridge University Press, 1993.
Moore, G. E. *Philosophical Papers*. London: Georg & Kegan Paul, 1965.
Morein-Zamir, S. & Sahakian, B. J. Pharmaceutical Cognitive Enhancement. In: Illes, J. & Sahakian, B. (eds). *The Oxford Handbook of Neuroethics*. Oxford: Oxford University Press, 2013. pp. 229-244.
Mouffe, C. *The Democratic Paradox*. London/New York: Verso, 2000.
Moyal-Sharrock, D. *Understanding Wittgenstein's* On Certainty. Basingstoke: Palgrave Macmillan, 2005.
Naess, A. The Shallow and the Deep, Long-Range Ecology Movement. *Inquiry*, 16 (1973, pp. 95-100.
Nature. Neuroscience.*Editorial* (The Ethical Neuroscientist). March 2008.
Nature. Neuroscience. *Editorial* (Ethical Neuroscience). February 2010.
Nelson, J. L. 'Unlike Calculating Rules'? Clinical Judgement, Formalized Decision-making, and Wittgenstein. In: Elliott, Carl. *Slow Cures and Bad Philosophers. Essays on Wittgenstein, Medicine and Bioethics*. Durham/London: Duke University Press, 2001. pp.48-69.
Nicolelis, M. *Made in Macaíba*. São Paulo: Editora Planeta do Brasil, 2016.
Noddings, N. *Caring. A Relational Approach to Ethics & Moral Education.* Berkeley: University of California Press, 2013.
Nussbaum, A. M. *Pocket Guide to the DSM-5 Diagnostic Exam*. Arlington: American Psychiatric Publishing, 2013.
Nussbaum, M. C. *Creating Capabilities*. The Human Development Approach. Camb/Mass.: The Belknap Press, 2011.
O'Neil, O. *Towards Justice and Virtue. A Constructive Account of Practical Reasoning*. Cambridge: Cambridge University Press, 1996.
O'Neill, O. *Autonomy and Trust in Bioethics*. Cambridge: Cambridge University Press, 2002.
Oliveira-Souza, R. &Moll, J. The Moral Brain: functional MRI Correlates of Moral Judgment in Normal Adults. *Neurology*. 54(Suppl.3), 2000.

Parfit, D. *Reasons and Persons*. Oxford: Oxford University Press, 1984.
Parfit, D. *On What Matters* (2v.) Oxford: Oxford University Press, 2013.
Partridge, B. &Lucke, J. & Hall, W. A Comparison of Attitudes Toward Cognitive Enhancement and Legalized Doping in Sport in a Community Sample of Australian Adults. AJOB *Primary Research*. V. 3, N.4, Nov. 2012, pp. 81-86.
Pellegrino, E. &Thomasma, D. *A Philosophical Basis of Medical Practice. Toward a Philosophy and Ethics of the Healing Professions*. New York/Oxford: Oxford University Press, 1981.
Pellegrino, E. &Thomasma, D. *For the Patient's Good. The Restoration of Beneficence in Health Care*. New York/Oxford: Oxford University Press, 1981.
Pellegrino, E *et al.* (eds.) *Transcultural Dimensions in Medical Ethics*. Maryland: University Publishing Group, 1992.
Pellegrino, E. &Thomasma, D. *The Virtues in Medical Practice*. New York/Oxford: Oxford University Press, 1993.
Pellegrino, E &Thomasma, D. *Helping and Healing. Religious Commitment in Health Care*. Washington: Georgetown University Press, 1997.
Persons, I.& Savulescu, J. *Unfit for the Future. The Need for Moral Enhancement*. Oxford: Oxford University Press, 2014.
Pessini, L.*et al.* (eds.). *Ibero-American Bioethics: History and Perspectives*. Dordrecht: Springer, 2010.
Pessini, L. &Bachifontaine, C. P. *Problemas Atuais de Bioética* (9thed.). São Paulo: São Camilo/Loyola, 2010.
Pontius, A. Neuro-ethics of 'Waking' in the Newborn.*Percept Mot Skills*, 37, 1973. pp. 235-245.
Potter, V. R. *Bioethics. Bridge to the Future*. New Jersey: Prentice-Hall, 1971.
Potter, V. R. *Global Bioethics*. Building on the Leopold Legacy. East Lansing: Michigan State University, 1988.
Quine, W. V. O. *From a Logical Point of View*. Nine Logico-philosophical Essays (2 ed.). Cam./Mass.: Harvard University Press, 1999.
Rachels, J. Active and Passive Euthanasia. In: Baird, Robert & Rosembaum, Stuart. (eds.) *Euthanasia: The moral issues*. Buffalo: Prometheus Books, 1989. pp.45-60.
Rachels, J. *The Elements of Moral Philosophy*. Boston: McGraw Hill, 2007.
Racine, E. *et al*. fMRI in the Public Eye. In: Farah, M. J. (ed.) *Neuroethics. An Introduction, with Readings.* Camb./MA: MIT Press, 2010. pp.185-190
Racine, E. Neuroscience and the Media: Ethical Challenges and Opportunities. In: Illes, J. & Racine *et al*. Can Neuroscience Contribute to Practical

Ethics? A Critical Review and Discussion of the Methodological and Translational Challenges of Neuroscience of Ethics. *Bioethics*. 31(5), 2017. pp.328-337.

Sahakian, B. (eds). *The Oxford Handbook of Neuroethics*. Oxford: Oxford University Press, 2013. pp.783-802.

Ragan, I. & Bard, I. & Singh, I. What Should We Do about Student Use of Cognitive Enhancers? An Analysis of Current Evidence. *Neuropharmacology*. Jan (2013) 64:588-95.

Railton, P. *Facts, Values, and Norms*. Cambridge: Cambridge University Press, 2003.

Ramsey, P. *The Patient as Person. Explorations in Medical Ethics*. New Haven/London: Yale University Press, 1977.

Rauscher, F. Kant's Moral Anti-Realism. *Journal of the History of Philosophy*. (3) 40, 2002, pp. 477-99.

Rauscher, F. Realism and Anti-Realism in Kant's Meta-Ethics: A Reply to Professor Dall'Agnol. In: Tonetto, M.*et al.*(eds). *Investigações Kantianas I*: um Debate Plural. Florianópolis: Funjab, 2012. pp.31-43.

Rauscher, F. *Naturalism and Realism in Kant's Ethics*. Cambridge: Cambridge University Press, 2015.

Rawls, J. *A Theory of Justice*. Cambridge/Mass.: Harvard University Press, 1999.

Rawls, J. *Political Liberalism*. New York: Columbia University Press, 1993.

Rawls, J. *Justice as fairness*. A Restatement. Cambridge/Condon: The Belknap Press, 2003.

Resnik, D. *The Ethics of Science*. London/New York: Routledge, 1998.

Rolston III, H. Caring for Nature: From Fact to Value, From Respect to Reverence. *Zygon*, v.39. 2004. pp.277-302.

Roskies, A. Neuroethics for the New Millennium. *Neuron.* 35(1), 2002, p.21-23.

Ross, D. *The Right and the Good*. Indianapolis: Hackett, 1988.

Ryle, G. *The Concept of Mind*. London: Penguin, 1990.

Sandberg, A. &Savulescu, J. The Social and Economic Impacts of Cognitive Enhancement. In: Savulescu, J.*et al.* (eds.). *Enhancing Human Capacities*. Oxford: Oxford University Press, 2011. pp.92-112.

Savulescu, J. & Bostrom, N. (eds.) *Human Enhancement*. Oxford: Oxford University Press, 2009.

Savulescu, J.*et al.* (eds.). *Enhancing Human Capacities*. Oxford: Oxford University Press, 2011.

Savulescu, J. Bioethics: Why Philosophy is Essential for Progress. *Journal of Medical Ethics*, v.41, 2015. pp.28-33.

Sharpe, V. A. & Faden, A. I. *Medical Harm*. Historical, Conceptual, and Ethical Dimensions of Iatrogenic Illness. Cambridge: Cambridge University Press, 1998.

Shue, H. *Basic Rights*. Subsistence, Affluence, and U.S. Foreign Policy. Princeton: Princeton University Press, 1980.

Singer, P. *Practical Ethics*. Cambridge: Cambridge University Press, 1993.

Slote, M. *From Morality to Virtue*. Oxford: Oxford University Press, 1995.

Stanley, J. *Know how*. Oxford: Oxford University Press, 2011.

Stein, Z. *et al*. Ethical Issues in Educational Neuroscience: Raising Children in a Brave New World. In: Illes, J. & Sahakian, B. (eds). *The Oxford Handbook of Neuroethics*. Oxford: Oxford University Press, 2013. Pp. 803-822.

Stewart, S. *et al*. (eds) *Patient-Centered Medicine*. Transforming the Clinical Method. London/New York: Radclife, 2014.

Suhler, C. & Churchland, P. The Neurobiological Basis of Morality. In: Illes, J. & Sahakian, B. (eds). *The Oxford Handbook of Neuroethics*. Oxford: Oxford University Press, 2013. pp. 33-58.

Svenaeus, F. Wittgensteinian Perspectives in Bioethics. (review) *Medicine, Health Care and Philosophy*. V.4, 2001, pp.97-9.

Syngh, I. Not Robots: Children's Perspectives on Authenticity, Moral Agency and Stimulant Drug Treatments. *Journal of Medical Ethics*. V.39, 2013, pp.359-366.

Syngh, I. & Kelleher, K. The Case for Clinical Management of Neuroenhancement in Young People. In: Chatterjee, A. & Farah, S. *Neuroethics in Practice. Medicine, Mind, and Society*. Oxford: Oxford University Press, 2013. pp. 16-34.

Swaab, D. *We Are Our Brains: a Neurobiography of the Brian, from the Womb to Alzheimer's*. New York: Spiegel & Grau, 2014.

Swanson, J. M. *et al*. Attention Deficit Hyperactivity Disorder: Defining a Spectrum Disorder and Considering Neuroethical Implications. In: Illes, J. & Sahakian, B. (eds). *The Oxford Handbook of Neuroethics*. Oxford: Oxford University Press, 2013. pp. 309-340.

Takahaski*et al*. Neural Correlates of Human Virtue Judgement. *Cereb Cortex*. (18), 2008.

Toulmin, S. *The Place of Reason in Ethics*. Chicago: University of Chicago Press, 1986.

Toulmin, S. How Medicine Saved the Life of Ethics.In: Jecker, Nancy *et al*. (eds). *Bioethics. An Introduction to the History, Methods, and Practice*. Sudbury: Jones and Bartlett Publishers, 1997. pp. 25-34.

Tugendhat, E. *Traditional and Analytical Philosophy*. New York: Cambridge University Press, 1976.

Tugendhat, E. *Problem der Ethik*. Sttugart: Reclam, 1988.

Tugendhat, E. *VorlesungenüberEthik*. Frankfurt am Main: Suhrkamp, 1994.

Tugendhat, E. *Egocentricity and Mysticism*. An Anthropological Study. New York: Columbia University Press, 2016.

United Nations. *The International Drug Control Conventions*, ebook available here: https://www.unodc.org/documents/commissions/CND/Int_Drug_Control_Conventions/Ebook/The_International_Drug_Control_Conventions_E.pdf<access 05/02/2019>

Urban, K. R. & Gao, W. J. Performance Enhancement at the Cost of Potential Brain Plasticity: Neural Ramifications of Nootropic Drugs in the Healthy Developing Brain. *Frontiers in Systems Neuroscience*. Vol. 8, Art. 34, 2014. pp.1-10

Veatch, R. *A Theory of Medical Ethics*. New York: Basic Books, 1981.

Vidarte, V. S. Reflexiones Wittgensteinianas. Reseñadel libro *Seguir Regras* de Darlei Dall'Agnol. *Pasajes*. V.40. 2012-3. pp.130-137.

Waldron, J. (ed.). *Theories of Rights*. Oxford: Oxford University Press, 1995.

Wall, F. *The Age of Empathy: Nature's Lessons for a Kinder Society*. New York: Three River Press, 2010.

Widdows, H. *Global Ethics. An Introduction*. Durham: Acumen, 2011.

Wildes, K. *Moral Acquaintances. Methodology in Bioethics.* Notre Dame: University of Notre Dame Press, 2000.

Wilkinson, D. *Death or Disability? The 'Carmentis Machine' and Decision-Making for Critically Ill Children.* Oxford: Oxford University Press, 2013.

Williams, M. *Problems of Knowledge*. A Critical Introduction to Epistemology. Oxford: Oxford University Press, 2001.

Wisnewski, J. *Wittgenstein and Ethical Inquiry. A Defense of Ethics as Clarification*. London: Continuum, 2007.

Wittgenstein L. *Werkausgabe in 8 Banden*. Frankfurt am Main: Suhrkamp, 1968.

Wittgenstein, L. Lecture on Ethics. *Philosophical Review*.V.74, 1965.

Wolf, S. *Feminism & Bioethics. Beyond Reproduction*. New York/Oxford: Oxford University Press, 1996.

Zak, P.L. *The Moral Molecule*. The Source of Love and Prosperity. New York/London: Penguin, 2012.

Zangwill, N. Against Analytic Moral Functionalism. *Ratio*. XIII, 3 (2000), 275.

Zimmerman, M. *et al*. (eds.) *Environmental Philosophy. From Animal Rights to Radical Ecology*. Upper Saddle River: Pearson, 1993.